Morgan 41

Morgan 41

Bob Erlich

ISBN 0966974956
EAN-13 9780966974959

Acknowledgements

I wish to thank all my friends in the great island nations of Trinidad and Tobago and The Bahamas for their kindness and generosity, the true inspiration behind this effort.

To Philip and Brian

Prologue

Growing up in Miami during the 1960's and 1970's it was impossible not to have been influenced or exposed to illegal drugs. It was just a fact of life in those days; with the sheer volume of the stuff flowing through the area, you were bound to run into it somewhere, even if you were not actively seeking it. I cannot remember any party I attended during that period where someone did not have a "joint," a "bong," a "line," or a "lude" at the ready, there for the taking and sharing like it was candy. "Spiking the punch bowl" used to be the big thing at teenage parties in Miami in the early 1960's, but by the end of the decade, it was almost a given that half the attendees at any party would be "stoned" out of their minds and several might also be "tripping."

Towards the end of the '60's and throughout the '70's we noticed a consequence of the over-abundance of drugs that as early teens we never thought much about. That consequence was the public explosion of violence that had previously been part of the shadow world of illegal drugs, something you just did not see as an every-day occurrence. Along with the rapid expansion of consumption came a huge surge of cash, which was immediately accompanied by a tremendous spike in violent crimes.

Such things came to my attention in the late 1960's and early 1970's as I worked my way through school. One of my many menial jobs in those days was as a maintenance man at an apartment complex near Miami International Airport. This complex was a very trendy spot in those days and was home to a collection of interesting characters, from go-go dancers at local clubs to Miami Dolphins football players. The complex management hosted free-wheeling parties on many a Friday afternoon, and a veritable smorgasbord of drugs was available for anyone who wished to partake. I never knew there were so many different types of LSD ("acid") - "purple micro-dot," "clear micro-dot," "purple haze," brown, white, "orange sunshine," "window pane," "red barrels," and many others. It all seemed pretty harmless at the time.

But one of the guys I worked with was a heroin addict. I'd never seen heroin and had little knowledge of it before "Craig" and I worked together, but I realized quickly that it was a killer. He was a "junkie," a painfully thin man with his arms and legs laced by needle tracks, evidence of his habitual abuse and addiction. He'd been to the methadone clinic and tried to switch but couldn't get the same high as he could with the "junk," so he just continued down the dead-end road he was on with no hope of escape.

I'd like to think he was eventually able to kick the habit, but the reality is that he probably didn't.

It was at about this time, in 1972 or '73 I think, when "coke" became very popular in Miami and supplanted heroin as the hardcore addict's drug of choice. It was so openly used and shared, and so cheap at the time that I can remember being offered "snorts" and "lines" at rock concerts by total strangers. Other drugs have come and gone or stayed popular for various generations - marijuana, heroin, LSD, mescaline, hashish, amphetamines ("speed"), PCP ("angel dust"), have all played their part through the years. Now, insidious chemicals such as methamphetamine and crystal meth are as prevalent in social gatherings as marijuana and LSD were decades ago, but with the ability to corrupt and destroy lives much more quickly and efficiently.

Regardless of all that came before and has happened since, what is clear is that cocaine in its various forms and methods of use/abuse has been and is still king. John DeLorean was accused of using it to help save his car company, John Belushi died from an overdose of it (in combination with heroin - a "speedball"), and even former Washington D. C. mayor Marion Barry fell victim to its lure. People in all walks of life and every imaginable profession have destroyed themselves and their families for it. Cocaine has proven to be an equal opportunity corrupter.

My world view relative to illegal drugs continued to expand rapidly in the 1970's as I personally witnessed the consequences of the drug trade. For me, it's as clear now as it was then - that the use of illegal drugs has had a devastating effect on the developed world for decades and despite all our efforts to the contrary, it continues to plague us. In the developed world we spend billions of dollars, pesos, euros, yen, yuan, etc. every year in a nearly futile attempt to staunch the flow of illicit drugs and eradicate their use. This is not news to anyone now, but in the early 1970's it was not commonly discussed by the public. Increasingly, our prisons have been filled with purveyors and users alike, criminals who steal to feed their habits, murderers who kill to defend their sales on a street corner or in an entire city.

But there is another facet of this problem that we are only now coming to grips with in a public way, although law enforcement has been struggling with it for many years. This need, this un-ending demand and craving for cocaine has changed not just the developed world, but the developing world in ways no one could have imagined in the 1950's and '60's. While we in the developed world squander our financial and human resources on its consumption, the developing world is locked in a life and death struggle for survival with the suppliers and purveyors of the product. We now bear witness to the ugly side of this struggle daily, on the evening news, online, or in the print media. Fortunately for now, we are rarely impacted directly by the horror and level of violence routinely visited upon the indigenous populations of many countries in Latin America and the Caribbean. US law enforcement agencies have been and still are heavily involved in these countries, working with local and federal governments in an attempt to win a nearly unwinnable war.

And there is no mistaking it - war is what is happening. Wars are literally taking place between governments and the heavily-armed narco-traffickers, criminals who often cloak themselves in illegitimate political causes and commit unrestricted acts of terrorism. The resulting violence overflows on a regular basis into the daily lives of average people who are just trying to get by. There is no doubt about what is occurring down South. It's truly a fight for survival, the rule of law against the certain insanity of anarchy and death.

Drug abusers today, especially in developed countries, are directly supporting this terrible war of attrition with every purchase they make. These consumers have a direct hand, a link to all the murders, mayhem and corruption that we see in the news media every day. Every line, every rock, every gram they use can be directly traced to the violence and corruption. This still profligate consumption is making the world a worse place for us all. If folks who consume illegal drugs don't understand this then they are just lying to themselves, their families, their friends, their employers, the people who count on them, the people who look up to them, and the people who love them. The only way we will truly end this heinous cycle fostered by consumption is to stop consuming the product. Once consumption dries up the market will cease to exist.

Failure by the developed world to end this irresponsible consumption of illegal drugs will condemn us all to a dismal fate. Soon, very soon, we will no longer be able to keep the violence and corruption at arm's length, off in some other country where they don't speak English as the native language. It will arrive one day in a shocking and very public way, and we will no longer be even marginally protected by our borders. As in the old adage about dispersing the problem "chickens," mark my words my friends, one day those "chickens" will come home to roost. Maybe in your neighborhood, maybe even on your own doorstep. When once we could claim blithe ignorance to the consequences of recreational drug use simply because we were in the nascent stages of the "information age" and perhaps really didn't know, we can no longer claim such ignorance. For all users of illegal drugs, the time of reckoning has come; things will only get worse from here unless we stop this ourselves.

So in the final analysis that's really the moral of this story: if you get involved with illegal drugs, you will be doing illegal things with bad people. Such acts have consequences, and it is a tale that never ends well for anyone. Don't forget it.

Chapter 1

"Donald, do you actually *know* where we're going?"

"Yes. Now stop worrying and just steer. Steer a course of three forty degrees, just west of north and we'll be there soon."

The *Madeleine* continued north along the bank, staying close to the shallow sand bars and low islands that dotted the area north of Andros. The boat was steady in the wind but the swells made it roll to port, putting the deck at an angle and adding to their stress. At least the weather was fair and there was a good wind for sailing, so they didn't have to go north using the small Yanmar engine that came with boat.

"Ok, I see the main island," said Donald. "According to the chart we still need to steer north or we'll ground in the sand shoals." He moved down to the wheel and showed his wife the map.

"See here, we'll need to stay between these patch reefs and the island. I'll stay on the bow and spot for you. You just steer where I tell you to."

Madeleine frowned. "Why do you have to act like *Captain Bligh*? I'm not your galley wench."

"Look, I'm just trying to get us there safely," he said, clearly agitated. "And by the way, do I have to remind you why we're doing this?"

"No," she said, pouting. She was unhappy with the situation but she had to agree, there was little else they could do.

They sailed on until the low sand dunes of the main island were clearly visible. The first dune line was covered with Australian pines which obscured the interior of the island as one looked west. No other boats were visible at anchor out in the sand shoals east of the shore, nor in the big tidal channel at the south end.

"Let's put in over there," said Donald, pointing to a spot opposite the middle of the island. "I'll get the forward anchor out. Turn her into the wind when I tell you."

He ran up to the bow and lowered the heavy Danforth anchor to the water.

"Ok, now," he yelled, and Madeleine steered her namesake to starboard and into the east wind. The mainsail went slack and the Genoa fluttered and flapped as the boat came around. Donald let the anchor drop as the boat slowed to a crawl and then allowed the west drift to set them up.

"Looks like we caught in a patch of grass," he yelled back.

Madeleine waved and moved up to lower the mainsail. Donald lowered the Genoa and tied it off securely before he went back to help his wife.

"I've got it," he said, taking over the task of securing the mainsail. Madeleine went into the cabin and quickly reappeared with a couple of bottles of Kalik beer, chilled down by the large Coleman cooler.

"Here," she said, handing her husband an opened bottle. "I thought we could use one after that trip."

"Thanks. Yes, it's a really good idea. I'm parched." He took a large gulp and sat back under the Bimini top.

"Now what?" she asked.

"Now we wait."

Madeleine was nervous, almost jittery in anticipation of the rendezvous. She hated this part of the trip, but she hated more the fact that their vacations had become something unpleasant, even ugly. She thought about the times they'd been out as a family, happier times when everyone just enjoyed being together and they had no daily worries or concerns except for where to find the lobsters for dinner that night.

"I'm going below to get the gun and get everything ready," said Donald. "Call me if you see anything. Take these." He handed her the binoculars.

She accepted them silently and watched him disappear into the cabin. Madeleine sat back and stretched her legs out on the seat cushion. The breeze was cool on her face, so she removed her hat and let the wind blow through her strawberry blond hair. The sound of the waves lapping against the hull was comforting, and she soon dozed off.

"Maddy, Maddy wake up!" Donald's voice sounded

urgent and shocked her back to consciousness. "Didn't you see them? What's the matter with you?"

"I'm sorry, I must have fallen asleep. Are you ready?"

"I think so. We're set up below. Here, put this under the cushion, in case we need it." He handed her the Ruger Redhawk .357 magnum revolver and she held it like it was a dead animal.

"I hate this thing," she said, shoving it under the rear cushion.

"Ok, I need to grab the lines. Remember stay cool and let me do the talking."

The roar of the three yellow Donzi Z-33 Crossbows was deafening as they approached the sailboat from the south. Donald had lines tied to his port and starboard cleats and was standing on the starboard side, ready to receive their "guests." The boats slowed to near idle as they approached, reducing their wakes to gentle rolls. Donald could see that each boat had two men this time instead of the three he'd seen on previous occasions. The lead boat came along side and he tossed the starboard line to the guy in the passenger's seat. The shirtless young kid pulled them close while the driver put the rumbling engines in neutral. The second boat copied the first but on the port side, and Madeleine noticed the third boat remained a short distance away, with its sharp bow pointed south.

"Welcome," said Donald, extending a hand to the driver. The guy jumped on board the sailboat and smiled.

"So you are the guy?" said the driver in a heavy

Spanish accent. He tilted his baseball cap up to get a better look at Donald.

"Yes, I'm the guy. Can we get started?"

"Sure, sure." The driver waved back to his young companion. "Hey, Calisto, let's go. Move the shit." He turned back to Donald and smiled, exposing his tobacco-stained teeth.

"So, you no offer me a drink?"

"Oh, sorry. Maddy, can you get the "captain" here a drink? And bring one for each of his men, would you?"

Madeleine said nothing but went to the cabin to retrieve some more beer. She was relieved not to have to be out there while everything was going on, but she also didn't want to be trapped in the cabin when the loading started, so she hurried and brought four cold beers to the deck.

The two passengers had begun shifting small burlap sacks from the cabins of the Donzi's onto the deck of the sailboat. The other driver began moving the sacks into the cabin, placing them below the floor panels in the main bunk area and inside the wall panels of the galley and outside bunk. It took about twenty minutes to completely unload the powerboats and load the sailboat, but soon the men were done with the chore and ready to enjoy their cold beers.

"Ok, we go now," said the captain. "Have a nice day."

He flashed his brown teeth again and climbed back into the driver's chair of his boat. The passengers untied their lines and both boats rumbled to life.

"We see you in Miami in two weeks," he called out.

Donald waved and the two boats rumbled out slowly towards their waiting companion. When they were safely clear of the sailboat, the three Donzi's roared to life and shot back towards the south. In moments they were out of view and soon, the sound of their engines had blended with the calm lapping of the waves against the hull of the *Madeleine.*

"Thank God that's over," said Madeleine.

Donald coiled the lines and stowed them in the storage locker. "I told you, the more we practice, the easier it gets."

"I know, but it still scares me. Look at what happened to Don Aronow. I don't want you to end up like that."

Donald gave his wife a hug, the first real sign of affection she'd seen from him since they left Nassau. "Don't worry, it's a piece of cake now. I'm going below to make sure all the hatches and panels are secure. We can spend the night here and then cruise over to Marsh Harbour like we planned."

He disappeared below and Madeleine sat back again against the rear cushion. Her stress level had definitely dropped, and she was finally able to relax and begin to enjoy the trip. She would worry about making dinner in a couple of hours. Right now, relaxation was on the menu.

After a short nap, Madeleine went below to check on the supplies. *Unless Donald catches something we can eat, I'm cooking out of cans tonight,* she thought. "Donald," she called up to him. "Any luck yet."

"I've had a couple of bites. We'll see what happens. By the way, what did you do with the gun?"

"I think it's still under the back cushion. Why?" She

thought she heard some tension in his voice.

"No, reason. Just want to make sure we don't forget where it is."

Madeleine did not like the sound of that. She poked her head out of the cabin and looked at her husband. "Donald, what's wrong?"

"Well, it looks like our friends are coming back," he said, staring south into the fading afternoon light. The sun was going down behind the trees on the island and long shadows flowed across the water towards them.

She came up on deck and grabbed the binoculars to have a look. "I don't know," she said. "You have a look." She handed him the binoculars and he stared intently at the rapidly approaching boats.

"Something's different," he said with a hint of alarm. "Looks like there is another boat with them this time. Well, let's find out what they want. The sooner we get done with these guys, the better."

Donald put his fishing pole down and once again tied his lines to the cleats. The sound of the boats grew from a buzz to a roar as they approached, and he could see there was a different group of people on the Donzi's than before.

"Maddy, better hand me the gun," he said.

§

"Excuse me. I'm sorry to interrupt but I'm looking for Mr. Eli Rose."

"You found him," Eli said, standing to greet her.

Vicente leaped from his chair and bowed, offering her the seat. She smiled and sat down with Vicente standing stiffly beside her, inspecting her clothes. He gave Eli a wink, as if to say that they would probably make a lot money on this job, for a change.

"So, Miss.............."

"McHenry. Josephine McHenry. You can call me Jo."

"So, Miss McHenry, how can we help you?" Eli smiled expectantly but without emotion.

"Well," she hesitated, looking askance at Rita and Vicente. Rita hopped up from her chair and excused herself, closing the door behind her. "Well," she repeated, "I need some help finding two people."

"I don't wish to be impolite, by why don't you go to the police? They deal with this sort of thing all the time. They're really pretty good at it," Eli said, trying not to be impatient with her. *It's a game*, he thought. *No truth here. What does she really want?*

"They suggested I talk to you. They said you were the best man for this kind of job."

"Ok, great. I'll have to thank the Assistant Chief next time I see him for that glowing endorsement. So what kind of job is this that only I can do?" Eli was running out of patience.

"It's my mother and father. They took our boat out to the Bahamas three weeks ago and haven't returned. I can't find out anything and the police won't help because they say it's out of their jurisdiction. The Bahamian authorities say that there's no evidence of any crime and that Mom and Dad probably just wanted to get away from the rat race. But I think something *bad* has happened to them."

"I don't know, Miss McHenry," Eli sighed.

"Jo."

"Fine, Jo. This really isn't the type of work we do but I can assign my best man here, Vicente Amarón, to do some preliminary work on your case. Why don't you two discuss this in the conference room where you can have some privacy?"

Jo pouted and frowned like a scolded child. "I was told *you* were the best man, Mr. Rose."

"Sorry," Eli smiled, enjoying the opportunity to dump her off on Vicente, "but *he's* the best man we've got."

Vicente shook his head vigorously and smiled, returning the favor to Eli just like old times.

"No is true, *señorita*. I am sorry but Sr. Eli is the best. I am only the next best man."

Eli glared at Vicente and reconsidered as the girl began to explain again. After all, just one look at those legs was enough to put doubts in his mind. The slit in her dress exposed a thigh most men would kill just to *see*. Eli contemplated his decision. A *real* platinum blond. Maybe too good an opportunity to pass up. He shook his head to clear his thoughts, and refocused on business.

"Mr. Rose, is something wrong?" the girl asked impatiently. Jo stared uncomfortably over at Vicente for a moment as if he was the source of Eli's distraction, and then began her story again.

"I'll start from the beginning in case you missed something," she sighed. "Mother and Father always take their summer cruise about this time of year, and they're often away and out of contact for extended periods. Naturally, I thought nothing of the fact that they hadn't called for a couple of weeks until a few days ago."

Eli leaned back and put his feet up on the edge of his desk to take the stress off his lower back. "So why did you suddenly think something was wrong?"

The girl leaned forward slightly as if she wanted to whisper some secret detail about her life.

"My father's partner, Lloyd Taylor called and asked to speak to him. When I told him that he and Mother were still sailing, Lloyd threw a fit. He said that Father had told him he'd be back in Miami on Sunday, and to call him at home. Here it was Wednesday, and I knew something wasn't right."

"So maybe your father just blew off the office for an extra week and took the long way back," Eli interrupted.

"Not likely," insisted Jo wistfully. "His business has always been the first thing in his life. If Lloyd was expecting him back, he would have been back."

Eli glanced over at his intercom to make sure it was set to ON. Rita would catch everything at the other end and he could cross-check with her after the girl left.

"Sorry. Please continue," Eli added apologetically.

"The cruises my parents usually take last no longer than three weeks, and they almost always stay in the western Bahamas; Father knows the islands very well. That's why this doesn't make any sense." She opened her white Gucci handbag and pulled out a note pad with some names and numbers jotted across the top.

"Let's see - here it is. I decided not to wait, so I called the police first."

"And they told you to file a missing person's report

and call the Bahamian consulate," added Eli, expecting the usual response.

"Yes. How did you know?" she asked. The tall blond leaned forward, exposing a dangerous view of tanned cleavage down the front of her white Halston suit. Eli shot a look over at Vicente, who sat across from him. Vicente was filing his nails and sitting by passively, almost disinterested. But Eli knew differently.

"That's what I would say if I were them. Metro-Dade PD has no jurisdiction over there, so unless you have a few well-placed friends to run interference for you, you have to ask the questions yourself." Eli wrote a quick note to himself to call Phil Rabinowitz at Metro-Dade and have him check to see if a report had been filed with anyone at Missing Persons.

"So what did the consulate tell you?"

"Since you're so quick, I'm sure you already know," Jo shot back.

"Ok, I'm sorry I was out of line," Eli lied calmly. "Please go on."

She smiled a perfect smile, all those white teeth capped and polished to a high gloss. "Naturally, they suggested that my parents had been caught up in the spirit of the islands, and had just decided to stay a while longer. They basically ignored me, but said they'd run a routine inquiry through their main police offices in the area." Jo sat back in the black leather chair and stared out the window. "That didn't inspire a lot of faith, if you know what I mean."

Eli smiled artificially, hoping she would get to the point a bit quicker but Vicente beat him to the punch.

"*Señorita* McHenry, I know this is difficult time for you, and also that you must have a good reason for the visit."

"Yes, of course," she snapped, but Vicente had made his point. "My time is valuable these days, since I have had to step into Father's place with respect to the company. As I was saying, I received no help through the normal methods of inquiry, so I was about to start looking on my own when one of the detectives at the Miami-Dade County Police Department gave me your name." Jo stopped to read a note she'd scratched at the bottom of the pad.

The central air conditioning system in the office started abruptly and instantly carried the fragrance of Chanel No.5 through the room like a cloud of nerve gas. Even the normally implacable Vicente winced at its power.

"Here it is," she sighed. "Brickell Avenue Associates. Eli Rose, President. Professional security services, lost and found, miscellaneous low profile investigations. After he droned on about you for a few minutes I realized I *had* heard something about you, after all. Some mess in China, from what I recall. In any case, the detective said you were one of the best at resolving these kinds of problems, so here I am."

The girl shoved the note pad back into her bag and stared at Eli like a raptor measuring its prey. Her cold blue eyes never wavered, and Eli wasn't certain he'd even seen her blink. She looked like a mannequin from the woman's department at the Saks Fifth Avenue in Bal Harbour.

"Well Jo, despite what you seem to have heard

about us, this is still not really our line of work. Perhaps I can recommend a friend at the State Department...."

Jo slammed her white bag down on the desk an inch from Eli's feet.

"Shit! I knew it!" she shouted. "There can't be one man left in this town with balls. Alright, fine. I can see that I'm wasting your time. Sorry to have bothered you." She launched herself out of the chair and was half way to the door by the time Vicente had grabbed her elbow.

"Hold on, hold on," Eli said quietly. "I'm not about to prove my qualifications to you, but maybe we could spend a little more time trying to help you find a good direction to go in. Please sit down, relax. Would you like a coffee?" Eli yelled at the door, "Rita, get Miss McHenry, er, Jo a coffee, would you? How would you like it?"

"Black, no sugar," she said sharply. Jo sat back down in the oversized chair in a huff, looking like a scolded child. Rita quickly entered bearing the coffee and a sour frown. Vicente grinned and looked towards the floor so she wouldn't notice.

Rita handed the girl the large ceramic cup and was greeted by as insincere a smile as Eli had ever seen. It was abundantly clear from just a few short minutes Jo was used to getting what she wanted, without any questions and at the speed of light.

"Anything I can get you gentlemen?" Rita said sarcastically. The two men shook their heads no, so she turned briskly away, poking Vicente hard in the shoulder on her way out of the room. He immediately rubbed the spot but leaned forward a bit in anticipation that Jo would finally reveal the interesting aspects of her dilemma.

"Now Jo, you know there are several possibilities for why your parents might not have checked in on time," Eli began.

"Go on," she said curtly.

"Well, on the positive side, you may have read your parents wrong just this once. Maybe your father really has chucked it all, at least temporarily and decided to play "Fletcher Christian" for a while with your mother on some out of the way island. Or maybe he's on his way in right now - he had engine problems, or ran into some bad weather."

"Mr. Rose, the detective at the police department told me you were as sharp as they come. Should I start looking for some better advice, as well as a new investigator?"

"Ok, since you're not in the mood to be humored I'll spell out the negative side for you," Eli said, expecting a bad reaction. "There are three equally nasty alternatives, each one probably fatal. If you want to talk accidents, maybe they hit some bad weather that capsized them or tossed them into the drink. They might also have been run down by a tanker making the run through The Straits – happens once and awhile, but I know you'll tell me that your father was too good a sailor for either one of those, right?"

Jo just smiled through her perfect, clenched teeth. "Well, then there's the real bad stuff. Depending on where they went they could have been either unlucky or just downright stupid."

"What do you mean by that?" said the girl, offended

at the hint of such a possibility.

"What I mean is that maybe they went too close to the wrong island and were boarded by pirates, or they saw something they shouldn't have and were capped by some narco-traffickers." Eli expected her to jump at the thought but she stayed calm. Too calm, he thought.

Jo paused silently in thought for a moment, her ice blue eyes focused on the floor. "So, if what I'm telling you is an accurate measure of my parents patterns, particularly my father's, what you're telling me is that they are most likely dead." Her eyes stayed transfixed on the floor and Eli glanced over at Vicente, who stared intently at the tall blond.

"What I'm telling you is that *if* one of those things has happened, then yes, they are probably dead." Eli pushed back in the chair, unconsciously distancing himself from the emotion beginning to flow in front of him. The girl's stony exterior finally started to give way, and tears began streaming down her face and onto her spotless white suit. *Ok*, he thought, *that's the reaction we should see.*

"I see," she sobbed. "Excuse me," she pulled a monogrammed handkerchief from her bag and dabbed at her eyes.

Rita, hearing the change in tone, re-entered quietly and stood close by. "Can I get ya' somethin', honey?" she said, patting the girl's shoulder lightly.

"No, thank you. Now let's continue please. How do we find out if the worst has happened?"

"Well, the first thing we'd do, if this was our case, would be to pay a visit to the Royal Bahamian Defense

Forces and check up on any unusual goings-on in the area. *Señor* Amarón here would make some discreet inquiries through his friends here in Miami, and then we might work backwards from where they were last seen. Ask some questions in the islands, you know, that sort of thing."

"Oh I see," she said, clearing her eyes at last. "And how much would this kind of inquiry cost me?"

"Our normal fee on something as unusual as this is two thousand dollars a day plus expenses, with fifty percent down. That's regardless of the result, and our average term has been in the neighborhood of about twenty days per case. Figure about forty to forty five thousand." Eli expected that to take care of any doubts that Jo could afford the services of his Brickell Avenue Associates agency, but he was floored by the girl's answer.

"Fine," she replied smoothly. "But what does that buy me - your routine investigation and maybe a written summary at the end of the job? Sorry, but I'm used to a higher level of commitment from my employees than that, and since you don't presently owe me your loyalty, perhaps I can buy it." The long, muscular legs flashed across Eli's errant gaze again as she pulled a leather checkbook from her bag. Jo slid the cover from a gold Monte Blanc pen and began writing.

"Tell me if this gets your attention."

Eli shook his head and began to dismiss her bravado before she handed over the green paper.

"Listen, this isn't really an issue of money. We're just not really in this line of work, so no matter how much you offer, you simply can't buy....." Eli paused, dumbstruck by the number written on the check. He had to stop all other non-essential brain functions to process the figure, a number he could barely comprehend.

Jo took advantage of his temporary stupor to offer the same question to Vicente.

"Well, *Señorita* McHenry, what *Señor* Rose tell you is true - this no is the type of work we do."

Eli waved at Vicente in an attempt to cut him off, hoping he wouldn't go too far before he showed him the check.

"What *Señor* Amarón means is that normally, this type of work would be out of our line. In the event a client insisted in our involvement, we would probably have farmed-out most of the routine investigative tasks."

He passed the check to Vicente, who said under his breath, "Son of a bitch! *Mama mia,* Eli."

"However, in view of some recent openings in our schedule, I think we will have the time and resources available to handle this for you." Eli had to consciously think about whether or not he'd wet his pants during the few heart-pounding moments he first held the check.

"Fine," she smiled arrogantly. "I thought you might be more amenable under the right circumstances." The tall blond stood up and smiled, extending her hand.

"Thank you so much for your time today, Mr. Rose, Mr. Amarón." Vicente bowed and kissed her hand. "I will expect to hear from you soon regarding your work plan so that I can approve of how you are going to spend my money." She withdrew a perfumed business card from her bag and jabbed it towards Eli's face between two fingers.

"Certainly," he said, forcing a smile. He accepted the card as graciously as possible considering the dominance message she was sending. "I'll call first thing in the morning to arrange a meeting."

"Don't bother," she sniffed, turning towards the door. "I'm tied up in meetings all day tomorrow. However, I do expect to hear from you no later than Wednesday. After all, every wasted moment could mean not finding Mother and Father."

"Of course." Eli had to sit on his anger but the potential reward for prudency was staring him in face, so he swallowed hard again and kept smiling.

"A pleasure, gentlemen," said Jo as she floated out of the room. Her perfume wafted around them again, as if it was slapping the two men in the face for the rude images they conjured.

Rita was fuming by the time the office door closed and she sprang to her feet like a cat. "Eli, Vicente, what the hell are you two *bobos* doing? How could you let her treat you like that? Are you crazy or something?"

Her face was red and her dark eyes burned holes in Eli, but he didn't care. He and Vicente exploded with laughter, and they collapsed into each other's arms, patting themselves on the back with amusement. Eli reached out and tugged the reluctant Rita close to his side and shoved the check under her nose.

"Read it, my dear, and know the pleasure of the zeroes."

She looked at Eli as though he was two cards shy of a full deck, and grabbed the small piece of paper from his hand. "Eli, this.....this is no joke? This is real? IT'S REAL?" Eli nodded and smiled. "Oh my God," she gasped. "I can't......it can't......My God!"

"That's right, my little "Girl Friday," Eli said happily. That's an official McHenry-Taylor company check for one million dollars you're holding. I think it's Miller time."

Chapter 2

The sun looked particularly bright and the sky particularly clear the next day. It's funny how a little money will improve your outlook on life, and it's safe to say that a lot of money has the potential to improve it that much more. The financial independence the McHenry case would bring to Brickell Avenue Associates made the decision seem relatively straight forward, so on Tuesday Eli worked diligently to have a smooth plan to present to his new employer.

He developed a flow chart to make it all look impressive, even though the plan was uncomplicated; Eli would contact his friend in the RBDF and arrange for a visit while Vicente would run down leads in Miami. He particularly wanted more information about the McHenrys normal routines, so Vicente had already made plans to talk to their neighbors and yachting friends.

After he received word from the Bahamas, Eli would fly over and hire a boat to check the current trouble spots for any signs of recent activity. He believed from the start that if the McHenrys had been as competent with their boat as Jo had suggested then they must have run into some bad guys somewhere. The only question in Eli's mind was where, and could he prove it?

Vicente also expressed some concern about the authenticity of the check that Jo had so casually dropped on them, so he wanted to ask a friend of his at Barnett Bank to run through the McHenrys finances. Eli had learned well the lessons Vicente had taught him regarding outward appearances, so he instantly agreed with his suggestion. That part, Eli decided, would not be in the plan he'd show to Jo.

"Eli, call on line two for you. It's Vicente," said Rita sharply through the speaker phone.

"Ok, thanks." Eli punched the button and greeted his new partner. "So, Vicente, what do you have to tell me?"

"Well, we have help now from the nephew of my sister who work at the bank. He say he check in the personal and business history of this people. Now I go to the Hibiscus Island Marina to ask question of the people there. Maybe we get something of value from this."

"Sounds good to me. Keep me posted - I'll have the new cellular phone with me, so ring me if you come up with anything critical. See you soon." Eli tossed the handle into the receiver and tried to put the finishing touches on the chart. He was never much of an artist but it seemed like drawing a straight line was the most challenging thing he could have planned for the day.

His hand shook like he was holding a power drill rather than a pencil. Maybe it was the thought of just how much was riding on the outcome of the meeting.

"Rita, call Miss McHenry for me would you please," Eli said politely. The door burst open almost immediately as Rita dashed into his office.

"Look, just because everything seems to be going so good, don't think this is gonna' change our relationship any," she shouted, looking genuinely concerned.

"Damn, can't a guy be nice once and awhile? You've got a chip on your shoulder a foot long. Chill out a little." Eli looked up from the delicate operation he was performing, trying to extract some degree of sympathy for his effort at decency.

"Sure a *guy* can be nice; anybody but you. You know what happened six years ago when I let you get *too* nice. I swore then that this part of our relationship would never change again, and you know that's the condition you agreed to when I came back to work here. Now don't screw it up."

The hot little redhead was really serious this time, and Eli couldn't blame her. He could see that there was no use trying to explain that he wasn't the same guy she knew in the old days, that he'd never treat her that way again if he'd had another chance. But it was pretty clear that she'd never trust him in the same way as before, so Eli forced himself to fit the mold she expected and was comfortable with.

"Ok, then get the hell out of my office 'till I call for you," he shouted. "Can't a guy get any work done around here without every bimbo on the planet trying to bother him?"

"That's much better," she smiled. The little *Cubana* turned to leave but then stopped and leaned across the desk for a second. Her huge, pendant-shaped breasts hung loosely in her checkered blouse like ripe *papayas*, tantalizingly close but only a tease for Eli.

"Give me some time, boss," she whispered. "I need to get my feet back on the ground first and I can't handle this if you move too fast." Her dark eyes sparkled the way Eli remembered and she brushed his face smoothly with her palm. Then she slammed the morning edition of the *Miami Herald* down right in front of his nose and yelled, "Here's your damn paper!"

The loud impact of the rolled up paper startled Eli back to the present, and he would have thrown it at her if she hadn't fled the office so quickly. He was about to return to his work when he noticed a headline in the local news section by his friend Bill Sexton, the investigative reporter: "*Questions of Money Laundering Spur Federal Investigation at McHenry-Taylor.*" Eli was still staring, half mesmerized by the headline when the speaker phone buzzed again.

"Ok, Eli, I have Miss McHenry on the line."

"Sure, sure Rita," Eli said, distracted. "Tell her I'll call her back."

"What? You called her, asshole. Now pick up the damn phone!"

"Oh, yeah, right," Eli said sheepishly, and punched the button. "Miss McHenry, I wanted to see if you had some time today to review our work plan for the investigation."

The silence at the other end of the telephone signaled an unpleasant start to the conversation. The girl suddenly replied at full volume, "Mr. Rose, I assume you are neither stupid nor hard of hearing, but in case one of those misfortunes is true, I will repeat what I said in your office on Monday: I will be available Wednesday to discuss your work plan; call me to arrange a meeting. Why do you waste my time repeating what has already been agreed upon? Oh, and I think I instructed you to call me Jo?"

"I'm sorry Miss......"

"Jo!" she shouted into his ear. "What is it with you people, anyway? Why can't you people follow instructions? I asked that you call me Jo, and you insist on ignoring my wishes by calling me *Miss* McHenry. That's what the servants call me, and I'm sick of it. It's disingenuous crap!" She paused in silence for another long moment and then continued. "Why don't you come for lunch? We can eat in the garden today and enjoy the breeze. Perhaps the air will help us both think constructively."

What a bitch! Eli had to consciously stifle the thought lest it escape into the telephone. "Sure that sounds fine," he answered diplomatically. "How about eleven-thirty?"

"Yes, that will be fine. The chef tells me he has some fresh snapper straight from the boat. Will that do?"

"Just fine," Eli sighed, trying to survive without insulting her. "See you then." He hung up the telephone softly and thought, *The hell with you*! "what a bitch," he said aloud.

Eli's blood pressure was definitely high, because he could feel his pulse pounding in his head. Things like that wouldn't have bothered him as much twenty years ago, but now it was too much to just suck up quietly. His lack of patience just made his stomach twist in knots and gave him a headache. He really did need to see a doctor about his blood pressure. In the end, Eli reminded himself that his future, as well as the futures of Vicente and Rita, was riding on how well he did his job and how well he managed Jo McHenry.

"Now wait just a minute," gasped Rita as she opened the office door. "I had no idea I made you so angry. Eli, I didn't mean....."

"No, no," he interrupted. "I wasn't talking to you. I wasn't actually talking to anyone but myself. That woman is starting to drive me nuts the way she talks down to me. I hope I can hang onto my temper long enough for us to do this job." Eli rubbed his forehead and collapsed back into his chair.

"What the hell is it with her, anyway?"

"I don't know," said Rita sympathetically. She walked around behind the chair and began rubbing his temples in smooth, soft swirls.

"You need to relax and handle this one differently from the others, Eli. She sounds like the kind of woman who is used to having people jump just for her own amusement. I think maybe you and Vicente should switch around this time - let him take the girl while you do the background check." She stopped rubbing and patted her boss' shoulder.

"All I know is that we can't afford to lose this one,

no matter what she says. You have to find a way to work through this. It's not like it was in the old days, you know." Rita smiled and walked back to her desk to finish typing the work plan summary sheets. Eli shook his head, knowing Rita was right. He just had to figure out how he would keep from punching Jo's lights out when they met face to face.

§

Vicente fit into the upscale marina set in a way Eli could never hope to. His tan, weathered face and thin grey hair were now perfect counterpoints for his broad, insightful smile. Driving the same stunning Corvette convertible Eli had first seen him in nearly twenty five years ago, the distinguished looking *Cubano* played the part to the limit - retired, plenty of money, plenty of time, and no woman in his life. Whenever Eli wanted to infiltrate the Bal Harbour or Coconut Grove social circles, Vicente had been the choice.

Eli gave his old mentor free reign to carry out his part of the investigation the way he thought best. So in the bright, breezy morning air, Vicente was already on his way to the home of a friend that lived on Hibiscus Island. He had planned to visit Enrique Ramírez for some time anyway, but this was a perfect excuse. Though Vicente often tired quickly of Enrique's tales of his own magnificence, Vicente could put up with a day or two of it in turn for the introductions he needed.

The old Corvette sounded like a large bore Cummins marine engine in the quiet, hibiscus laden lanes of the island, but Vicente liked the way it announced his presence. He pulled up to the gate of his boyhood friend and rang the buzzer at the intercom.

"Yes, can I help you?" blared a voice from the over-amplified speaker.

"*Si*, er, yes. I am Vicente Amarón, here for to see *Señor* Ramírez."

"Thank you, sir," came the androgynous reply. Vicente climbed back into the idling car and coasted through the opening gates. He circled the drive and parked outside the front door as he usually did. The door was open by the time he reached the steps.

A cordial, yet indifferent young house maid greeted him and ushered him into the main living room. "Mr. Ramírez will be with you momentarily. Would you care for a drink sir?"

The pretty girl seemed interested enough in his well-being, so Vicente answered in Spanish, "Yes. I would like an orange juice, please."

The young girl never blinked, but replied in English, "Yes, of course, an orange juice. And would you like ice with that?"

"Yes," Vicente said in English, somewhat disappointed. He often tried to elicit a conversation in Spanish from the younger people he came into contact with, but while *Anglos* and *Cubanos* alike seemed to understand him, very few ever wanted to answer him in Spanish. Vicente just could not understand why not.

The house maid walked off swiftly and left Vicente alone in the cool room. He surveyed the contents and smiled at the thought of so much money. A small bronze by Rodin graced a modernistic chrome and glass table in the corner, and paintings by Dali, Picasso, and Miró adorned the walls. The north wall of the room was occupied by a large sliding glass door with a grand view of the Intracoastal Waterway and Miami Beach. The sculpted coral stone walkway that flowed away from the door led out to a large swimming pool and jacuzzi, and down to a dock where a sleek yellow *Cigarette* racer bobbed slowly in the waves.

Vicente's thoughts wandered and he didn't notice the girl return with his drink. "Here you are sir," she said politely. "Mr. Ramírez says you can come out to the pool when you're ready. He's finishing his morning swim."

"Thank you," said Vicente walking to the door. He sipped the cold juice and walked out onto the palm-shaded patio. The cool breeze was a perfect complement to his drink, and again he had to fight feelings of *déjà vu* from Cuba. Thoughts and dreams about the *Malecón* – they seemed to be coming more frequently these days, and the old man wondered whether that meant that his mind was failing or he was so homesick that nothing could quiet his desire to return before he was too old to do so.

He glanced over at the pool and could see Enrique gliding through the water with his head down. Vicente ambled over to a small collection of deck chairs and sat under the welcomed shade of a beach umbrella while Enrique calmly swam the last of his laps. The pear-shaped old man emerged from the pool wiping the water from his eyes, and waved over at Vicente when he could see who awaited him. Enrique's personal valet held open a terrycloth robe and then handed the plump little man a towel as the he returned to the house.

"Vicente, you old snake, it's so good to see you again." Enrique extended his hand and squeezed Vicente's warmly, slapping him on the back with the other hand. "How long has it been? One year? Two years?" He sat down and began to pour a glass of juice for himself from a cold pitcher that accompanied his breakfast.

"Too long, my friend," replied Vicente. "But I remember the last time I am here we speak only Spanish. You no speak Spanish any more here?" Vicente wanted to understand the phenomenon better and perhaps his old friend, now part of the change, could explain it in a way Vicente could comprehend.

Enrique ignored the question momentarily. "Can I offer you something more? Perhaps some melon, or fresh *papaya* from Mexico? They are not as good as the ones we had at home, but it is difficult to get them fresh, even from Mexico. The bastards like to pick them green so they last longer." He looked over the orange-pink fruit on his plate with disdain.

"They are not as sweet as ours were." Vicente waved off his offer, so Enrique continued. "So, you wish to know why I do not speak Spanish in this house. It's a good question, no? I can tell you very simply - it's about practice. I have to practice my English so that I can sound more *Anglo*."

Enrique didn't even wait for Vicente to ask him what he was talking about before continuing. "Look at this breakfast," he interjected disdainfully. "Decaffeinated coffee and fruit is all my doctors will allow me to have these days. After the heart problems last summer they have put me on a strict diet and exercise program. You know, nothing that enriches life, nothing that provides *El Sabor*, The Flavor. But still, I manage to have a good cigar from time to time."

"Enrique, what is happen to you? Are you *Cubano* or *Anglo*?," asked Vicente with a note of concern.

"*Amigo*, those days of clear separation between *Anglos* and *Cubanos* are over. Just look at how the young people act - they all want to be *Anglo* now. They all want to fit in, to make it in this country. Most of them were born *here*, not in Cuba, and they don't identify with Cuba - certainly not the Cuba that we knew."

Enrique sipped his juice and dried his face with a swipe of his hand.

"I do business with a different set of people than you do, and the people I do business with play golf and go to the yacht club with their second or third wives. I have to fit into that group if I don't want to be on the outside. So now I am trying to fit into the power structure of both worlds, and that is why we speak English in the house." He smiled and then said, "To be clear about this, it is my business to fit in. You see - English without an accent. What do you think?"

The words rang hollow in Vicente's ears, and although he understood what Enrique said clearly enough, he still could not agree.

"What a shame," Vicente exclaimed. He took a sip of his juice and stared silently, disapprovingly at

Enrique.

For his part, Enrique seemed satisfied with his explanation so he continued his soliloquy.

"Now my friends travel to Bogotá, and Caracas, as well as New York, Chicago, and London. I want to move in all these circles and this is the key to success in my business."

Vicente knew he was right, but would resist the change for himself until his last breath. His command of English had actually gotten *worse* over the past decade then it was in the 1950's and 1960's, mainly because he rarely dealt with English-only speakers since he stopped working for Murray Morgenthal. He wasn't happy about that, but accepted it as a function of growing old.

But in the upper end of the fashion business that Enrique dealt with, one needed to move in a variety of spheres in order to make the right connections, and seamless transitions from Spanish to English were a huge advantage. That was, in fact, why Vicente had come to visit him in the first place: not just for his contacts, but also because the McHenry-Taylor Group was perhaps the premiere design house in the southern United States. Enrique would naturally be in tune with the rumor mill that churned through the industry, and his contacts could provide valuable insight into the backgrounds and finances of the McHenry family.

"My old friend, I know you did not come all this way here to discuss my metamorphosis," said Enrique from the rim of his coffee cup. "What service can I offer you on this fine morning?"

"Yes, you are quite correct," said Vicente, switching to Spanish. "I have a job, Enrique. I am working again with Eli. We are making a routine investigation into the disappearance of Donald McHenry and his wife Madeleine in the Bahamas three weeks past. I was thinking that maybe you can provide some information on the health of the business, and maybe introduce me to some of the friends."

The plump little man smiled faintly and gently replaced his coffee cup on the table. He stood and walked briskly to the sliding glass door where his valet waited, and instructed him in an animated way to do something quickly. The man ran back into the house and Enrique returned to the table, but did not sit.

"Come with me, old friend," he answered in Spanish." We will have some things to discuss about this man McHenry."

The two men walked back into the house and Vicente followed Enrique into his bedroom. The valet had prepared the old man's clothes in the manner one would expect of an exclusive clothier, set aside with several possible combinations of shirts and ties to choose from. Vicente sat in a large rattan chair and breathed in the brisk aroma of sandalwood and musk spices that hung in the room. The warm accents of Florida pine and cypress graced the walls and floor, and the lazy breeze spinning off the ceiling fan reminded him of his own home in Havana, now long expropriated by Castro's government.

"I don't think I will wear a tie today, Tomás. Mr. Amarón has set a fine example with his open collar and casual slacks, so I think I will follow his lead."

"Very good, Mr. Ramírez," said the young man in English. He walked quickly to the closet and withdrew a selection of three casual shirts and trousers from which to choose, and Enrique grabbed the khaki's and a white Christian Dior short sleeve shirt.

"Good selection, sir," said Tomás rather mechanically as he began to replace the other offerings back in the closet.

"Tomás is interested in learning this business from me," said Enrique without warning. The old man looked admiringly at his young valet's rear. "He is from a fairly humble background and has offered his services as my valet in return for the introductions into the design business that I can provide him. We find this arrangement works quite well for now, don't we my young friend?"

Tomás chimed in, "Yes sir. Mr. Ramírez has been a great help to me so far. This fall, I will begin an apprenticeship with Alexander Julian, and perhaps by next summer I can move to Paris. Mr. Ramírez has been discussing the possibility with the house of Yves St. Laurent." The kid could not have been over twenty or twenty two years old, and to Vicente that seemed very young for these kinds of opportunities. He often wondered about Enrique's gender preferences. Obviously, along with his new-found lifestyle, Enrique was no longer concerned about how his sexual preferences were perceived.

As if to counter the thought in Vicente's wandering mind, Enrique added, "Tomás is a very talented young designer. He could just use some training from the more experienced houses and a few tips on managing his business relationships from me." The old man smiled weakly and continued dressing.

Tomás finished his work and exited the room in a rush. Enrique reached over to his nightstand and put on his Rolex President, grabbed his wallet and car keys and motioned Vicente towards the door.

"Let's take a ride, my friend, and I will tell you tales of this business that would make even Fidel blush."

Chapter 3

Eli had probably made the drive from his Brickell Avenue address to Venetian Causeway a thousand times, but it always seemed to relax him more than any other stretch of road in the city. Maybe it was the feeling of freedom he felt when he left the walled-in confines of Brickell and emerged at the Eternal Flame monument at Bayfront Park, like being reborn into the rare open stretch of downtown Miami that hadn't yet been completely swallowed by concrete.

Making the turn after the *Herald* building and squirting out onto the first bridge instantly transported Eli to another place and time, when the Miami of his younger days was the small town that so many people now wished it could be again. The old money islands of Biscayne Bay - the Venetian Islands, plus Star, Hibiscus, and Palm Island still retained the charm of old Miami in spite of the condominiums and infrequent new homes. Crossing those low bridges and embracing the unobstructed view of the bay always made Eli smile in a way he seldom did now.

The McHenry estate was tucked back off the road on the north end of Rivo Alto island, and Eli managed to drive past it the first time before he'd even realized it. The wrought iron gate was open so he drove into the short semi-circular drive and parked opposite the front door. The house was certainly unobtrusive from the front; long and low in tan, painted stucco, with green clamshell hurricane shutters, an orange, Spanish tile roof, and a narrow strip of grass they probably thought of as a lawn.

Eli rang the doorbell and waited impatiently in the steamy alcove of the entrance until the door opened with a rush of cool air. "Yes - can I help you, sir?," said the older gentleman, softly.

"My name is Eli Rose. I have an appointment to see Miss McHenry."

"Ah yes, Mr. Rose. We were expecting you fifteen minutes ago. Do come in." His less than subtle rebuke left Eli colder than the air conditioned entrance hall but he followed the guy silently into the main living room.

"Please have a seat. I will tell Miss McHenry you have arrived." The scarecrow-thin man didn't wait for any chance of reply and left quickly to get his employer.

Eli marveled at the vast expanse of leather furniture arrayed around the room. Surely an entire herd of cattle had perished in order to equip the place with its overly abundant seating. He laughed to himself at how all the rich people he'd ever met had decorated their houses in white. White leather furniture, white carpets, white window coverings, white paint on the walls. It gave him the impression of being inside a milk bottle and reminded him of times when his mother and father had visited well-to-do relatives in Bal Harbour. The things he remembered most about those visits were that the place was white from floor to ceiling, and that he was told not to touch anything for fear of leaving a smudge.

Maybe it was that subconscious scolding from his mother that made Eli fold his hands across the folder he held in his lap. That's how he was sitting when Jo McHenry strode into the room, her long white hair flowing out behind her like a regal robe. She was wearing a pair of white open-toed Oscar de la Renta sandals and a peach colored see-through sun dress, which allowed a tantalizing glimpse of her shapely form while retaining just enough modesty in the critical locations.

"Mr. Rose, good to see you again." Jo extended her hand and smiled politely. "You're a little late, but no matter. Shall we have lunch?" Before Eli could utter a word the leggy young girl answered for him. "Fine, let's go," she said.

Eli followed his new employer across the parquet floor to a small office that overlooked the bay and they sat in large leather chairs with big, soft cushions. The chef entered almost immediately and advised them of his midday offering.

"Miss Jo and Mr. Rose, good afternoon. Today I have prepared fresh grilled red snapper in a lime-garlic sauce with a mango-*habanero* chutney. As an accompaniment we have a cold lobster salad, deep fried yam sticks, and Andalusian gazpacho." The portly old fellow smiled as he spoke, obviously thrilled with his creativity and flair for the dramatic.

"For dessert, a fresh fruit plate composed of pineapple, *papaya*, and green melon slices with some nice fresh raspberries for color."

"Sounds great, Fredo," said Jo impatiently. "Thanks much."

"Oh, and might I recommend the Drouhin Mersault, Miss Jo?"

"Yes, yes," she said, becoming agitated. "That will be just fine. THANK YOU, FREDO."

The little Italian got the message loud and clear the second time and smiled, but left the room quickly. Jo rubbed her forehead in mock anguish and said, "He's my father's idea. So is Fredrick, the cold fish that greeted you when you arrived, and Francesca our housekeeper. Father has had them around forever and he loves the pomposity of it all."

"Well, I suppose you could get used to this kind of treatment," Eli said half joking.

"Maybe *you* could get used to it, but it drives me crazy," she shot back. "He decided that all the help had to have names that started with the letter "F." Jo leaned over the table and whispered, "If I had my way, I'd clear the place of all the "f-ing" hired help and just have a cleaning lady or two."

"Yes," Eli whispered back, trying to stifle a laugh. "A cleaning lady or two. That would work."

Jo sat back in her chair and a large shock of flowing platinum hair plummeted over her right shoulder. She pushed up the baggy sleeves of the dress and crossed her exquisitely long legs.

"Now, Mr. Rose, I know you didn't come here to discuss the vagaries of my domestic staff. You were supposed to bring a work plan for me to proof. Do you have it ready?"

Eli was again transfixed on those perfect legs, and had to catch himself to keep from looking like a jackass. He held up the expandable wallet folder he'd brought and she said, "Good. Let's get down to business. What's the first step?"

Fredrick appeared with the wine just at that moment and silently poured two very full glasses. Before they could taste the clear golden liquid he announced, "I have sampled the contents and have found them to be satisfactory." Eli shot a glance at Jo while they were lifting their glasses to drink, and when she saw his look of astonishment she nearly burst out laughing.

"Yes," she said, stifling a laugh. "I'm certain everything is great. Thank you Fredrick." She looked down and smiled into her glass as the stiff old man left the room. Finally, she could no longer contain her laughter and attempted to muffle the outburst in her cupped hands. "God, do you believe that?" she chuckled.

"Pretty amazing. But I'll tell you what's even more amazing," Eli said, seeing a chink in her armor.

"What's that?" she laughed, still amused by the stilted manner of her father's valet.

"You. That's the first time I've seen anything resembling a genuine smile cross your face since we met. I was beginning to think you were mad at the world. I can see now that when you smile like that, your whole face brightens. You could bring a lot of men to their knees with that smile."

Her mood and facial expression changed instantly from that bright, happy demeanor to a frowning, dark stare.

"Mr. Rose, I was warned about your reputation with the ladies so let's clarify something right from the start – you are in my employ, and nothing more. If you ever make a pass at me again, I'll throw you off this case so fast it will make your head spin. Do we have an understanding here?"

The venom in her voice was palpable and very clearly understood. "Sorry. I was only trying to pass on a compliment. You just seemed so genuinely happy and vibrant at that moment that I had to say something. It won't happen again." *Great!*, thought Eli. *Just what I need – another "Alpha female" for a boss*!

"See that it doesn't," she replied curtly. "And another thing – I'm not the happiest person in the world right now, as I'm sure you can well imagine. After all, that's why you're here. But I also have no trouble admitting that the second part of what you said has been only too true."

"You mean the part about bringing men to their knees?" Eli asked with feigned innocence.

"I don't know what it is about you men," she said. "You all sound so smooth at first, but you're all so weak when it comes right down to it. Maybe I'm just unlucky at love; I don't know. But I can definitely say that I haven't met a man yet that I couldn't wrap around my little finger."

Eli thought about pursuing the conversation further

but remembered her warning about getting too cozy. He refocused on the job at hand.

"Well, that's interesting. Now then, the plan is.........."

"What I mean to say is that men are all so transparent," she interrupted, continuing to drive the conversation. Jo was clearly plugged into some inner flow of consciousness and was reluctant to release the thought.

"Most of the men in my life have wanted only one of two things from me." She paused, expecting Eli to ask which two things, but he already knew what she was going to say. "It's either been my money or my body, "she sighed, as if truly perplexed.

"I'm sorry about that," Eli insisted, trying in vain to drag the conversation back to business.

"You're sorry?" shouted Jo. "How do you think I feel? All you weasely little wimps out there, squirming around trying to get into my bank account or my pants."

"Now hold on a minute," Eli said a bit angrily, offended by the remark. He was about to launch into a stout defense of all the men in the world just as Fredrick arrived with the gazpacho.

"Gazpacho," he said in a monotone, setting two small bowls down beside them.

"Wonderful," said Jo smiling broadly. "Thank you Fredrick. Well, I'm starving and this looks great. Let's eat." She brushed her white hair aside and began attacking the cold soup with vigor.

"Yeah, it looks great," Eli repeated curtly. "Now, what was that you just said about all of "us" men?"

Jo dropped her shoulders suddenly and sighed loudly. "Look, *you* tell me. What is it about men that makes them so dishonest? I mean, and here's a perfect example, I met this guy at a cocktail party that Father was sponsoring for new clients. He said all the right things to me, took me to all the right places, moved slow at the right times and fast when he should. Then surprise, surprise. I find out that the guy's married and he's only in it for a quick fling."

Eli sucked down a mouthful of the cold soup and said, "Ok, so the guy was a prick. But that doesn't mean that *all* of us are pricks."

The tall blond thought for a second and then said, "Yes, but that's not the point."

"Well, then, what is the point?"

She sighed again. "Well, why didn't he just tell me that in the first place? I wouldn't have minded boffing him for a couple of months and just sharing a couple of laughs, but this guy *lied* to me, and that's what I can't understand and cannot tolerate."

"Miss McHenry......"

"Jo!"

"Right, sorry. *Jo*, you're diving into the world of the unknown here. Men and women have been asking themselves these same questions since before language developed beyond a grunt, and I haven't heard a reasonable explanation yet for why men and women can't tell each other the truth. Wouldn't it have just been easier to write the guy off as scum and move on to the next guy?"

She looked up from her soup for a second and appeared to grin just a little.

"You mean, you aren't going to try to make excuses

for your kind?"

"You can't make excuses for someone like him. It's too bad he turned out to be someone else but that's life. Get over it already and cut us men some slack. Cut *me* some slack and maybe we can communicate with a bit less friction."

Eli felt more like her psychoanalyst than the investigator she said she wanted. There was a ton of hostility in the girl's voice and he suspected there was more than just one failed tryst behind it.

"So," Eli said with a slow pause, "can we move on and get down to business?"

She smiled again but continued eating for a minute or two without speaking. Eli was sick of the game she was playing but was mindful of the huge check she'd handed him. *If she wants to confess to me for a year then it's her money*, he reasoned.

"So what's the plan?" she suddenly blurted out.

Finally! Eli felt the onset of a sharp sinus headache behind his right eye, a telltale stress response to her instantaneous mood swings.

"I have the plan here," he answered, rubbing his eye. He pulled out the flow chart and laid it on the table next to the soup bowls. "The first stage of the investigation will involve the usual official Q&A here and in the Bahamas. We'll follow that up with some "unofficial" contacts until we have a good lead that cross-checks."

"Sounds Ok to me," she said, studying the diagram. "And where do I come in?"

"I'm sorry?" Eli replied. His thoughts had wandered to the first visit he would have to make to Nassau to see his friend Leslie Robertson of the RBDF. "I'm sorry, what did you just say?"

"What I said was, where do *I* come in? What's my part? When do I get to be involved?" She looked at him with wide-eyed anticipation like a child about to start a game with friends. Eli had the impression she wanted him to point to the parts of the plan where a note would say, "Jo does this," or "Jo does that."

Eli shook his head and rubbed his eye again. The headache appeared to be worsening by the minute and he started to fumble around in the folder for the small bottle of aspirins he always carried just for times like this.

"Excuse me a second," he said grabbing a couple of the pills and quickly washing them down. *Why is it that every time I have a female employer she wants to get involved and then run the show?* he thought. Maybe he seemed like a sympathetic figure to them. He couldn't understand it.

"I'm sorry Jo, but I guess I didn't understand you at first. You said that you *want* to be involved with the investigation?" Eli's momentary confusion was interrupted by Fredrick and a tray of now unappetizing food.

"The snapper, Miss McHenry, Mr. Rose," said the old man with bland indifference. He carefully put the plates in front of them. "Do enjoy," was his emotionless offer.

"I'm sorry if I've somehow managed to give you the impression that you'd be directly involved with the investigation," Eli continued, "but that's not really part of the plan."

The girl stabbed the snapper aggressively with her fork and began chewing a large mouthful.

"Make it part of the plan," she replied assertively, partly muffled by the fish.

"I'm sorry but I see that you don't understand. Well, the fact is that I don't really have the time to escort you around during this phase of the investigation and in truth, it's really a pretty boring exercise. Perhaps...."

Jo threw her fork at her plate hard enough to make it bounce off and onto the floor.

"Fuck that!" she yelled. "Who the hell do you think you are, anyway? Now get something straight here, Mr. Rose. I'm paying your goddamn salary, and I'll do whatever I goddamn please, whenever I please. Do *you* understand me?"

She glared at Eli with her icy blue eyes and he realized that resistance was futile.

"Ok, Ok. There is a way for you to help out if you feel like you have to do something," Eli sighed, trying to limit the damage.

"*Want* to do something?" she growled. "*Want* to do something? Do I have to repeat what I just said, Mr. Rose? Are we clear about this or is there something in the words "fuck that" that you don't understand?"

She paused, her face and neck now flushed red with anger.

"And I'm not just talking about doing *something*. I'm going to be your shadow, Mr. Rose. I'll be with you every step of the way. If you don't want me to stop payment on that check, you'll work with me on this."

Eli's headache had not improved, and now his stomach was twisted into a knotted mess. He took a deep breath and walked over to the window to look at the bay. It always seemed a calming view in the past. He hoped the view would help him keep from saying something really stupid.

"Ok, Jo. It's your money at the end of the day. I'm only saying that based on my experience, our team will be far more effective and more likely to succeed without additional "help" from the outside. If you're determined to be part of this thing then there are some ground rules you'll have to follow. Agreed?"

"Fine," she hissed. "What?"

"First and most important, you're a passenger until or unless I ask you for your help."

"Ok, agreed. Next."

"Next, I ask the questions and manage the investigation."

"That sounds reasonable," she said, resuming her feeding frenzy with Eli's fork. "Just think real long and hard about how this is going to work with me in it, because the first time I get wind of you talking down to me or keeping things from me, you're out of a job. Understand?"

Eli marveled at how cold blooded she sounded, considering how warm blooded she looked. "Fair enough. So I guess I should tell you to expect to travel to Nassau tomorrow. We're going to visit a friend of mine in the RBDF."

Jo smiled for the first time since they'd started their lunch "meeting" and glanced up at him from the small pile of white bones on her plate.

"Just tell me when and where, and I'll be there."

Eli hoped Vicente was faring better than he was

with his part of the investigation. Eli wasn't looking forward to hearing Vicente laugh when he told him that Jo was going to be tagging along for the duration.

"Fine. Then be at the Bahamasair desk at Miami International at nine tomorrow morning. Bring some casual business clothes, a couple of bathing suits, some sandals and whatever toiletries you'll need for a week in a waterproof bag."

"Why a waterproof bag?"

"Well, once we leave Nassau we'll be going for a boat ride, and we're liable to get a little wet. And now I hope you'll excuse me – I've got to make a few changes to accommodate you. Thanks for the lunch."

Eli turned to go but the girl reached out and grabbed his arm, using it to pull herself out of her chair.

"Why don't you stay for desert. I'm sure it will be worth the wait." She smiled and made him think of all the times in his life that a line like that had been used to suggest something else. He shook his head and smiled politely.

"No thanks," he added. "Got to watch the waistline in my old age. Maybe some other time."

As he left the room Eli heard her say under her breath, "Asshole. What does he want, an engraved invitation?"

Eli almost turned around in mid step, but thought better of it and continued out to his car. As he drove back towards the office he decided to stop off at the *Herald* and visit Bill Sexton, the guy who wrote the investigative story on the McHenry-Taylor Group. If there was any truth to the rumor of money laundering at the company it definitely would have provided a good motive for the McHenrys to just "disappear." Vicente's background check and a run through their personal finances would give him a much clearer picture of the possibilities.

As far as Jo was concerned, Eli was determined this time to keep his mind from wandering off to topics other than business. Allowing himself to get emotionally involved with his female bosses hadn't worked well for him in the past, and he sensed something odd about this girl that made his skin crawl. Still, he suffered from the irresistible temptation that such beauty often engendered, his "sweet tooth" as he often referred to it. He hoped that this time his disquiet with the girl's motives would be enough to save him from his overpowering taste for sweets.

Chapter 4

"You don't have any idea how big a son of a bitch this guy McHenry is," said Enrique. He glanced away from the road to catch Vicente's reaction but as usual, there was none. The plump, balding little man continued driving his red Cadillac El Dorado briskly through the Collins Avenue traffic while looking over at Vicente, who watched only the neighboring cars.

"If he is in some kind of trouble I say good - screw him and his whore of a wife, too."

"Enrique, I know that you no say these things for no reason, so *por favor*, no to make this difficult." Vicente was impatient with Enrique's constant insults to the McHenry family, especially since he hadn't yet said anything incriminating about them.

"So you say this man is son of a bitch because he steal ideas from you and others; he break contracts; maybe he no like to make love to his own wife. Ok, so you no like him. But this is illegal?"

"No, *amigo*, obviously not. What I am trying to say is that this man has a bad history, understand? And I was hearing that his partner was preparing to sue him

for misappropriating money from the business."
Enrique began to speak more quietly, and his
expression became cold, serious.

"Now this man all of a sudden begins to have
financial problems, after twenty five years in the
business, and just as quickly he has a major infusion of
cash from an unknown "investor." So the IRS says wait
a second, Mr. McHenry, but I don't think this is so
kosher."

"So you say he hear about this investigation by
IRS?"

"*Si, amigo.* And not just IRS. A strong rumor has
been circulating about the Justice Department looking
into the source of the funds, that maybe they are from
Cali or La Paz or maybe even *Habana.*" Vicente
nodded and noted the turn to Bal Harbour.

"Today I am taking you to a party at the home of a
very influential *Anglo* called William Sandifer. He and
his wife are good friends of the McHenrys, and Mr.
Sandifer is also that bastard's personal banker. In this
way, perhaps you can determine the value of the check
the daughter gave you."

"*Gracias* for the opportunity, my friend, but you
have to help me with this."

Vicente's palms began to sweat slightly. In spite of
his outward appearance and demeanor, he was always
uncomfortable with this part of his job. Although he
was accustomed to insinuating himself into *Anglo* and
Latino society it was always just a *façade.* The society
he knew best, the one he could slip through without a
ripple was the one he'd left behind many years earlier.
He always knew what to say and how to act when he

was Morgenthal's man, his personal *caudillo*, his "strongman." He could handle the guys from New York, Chicago, and Las Vegas with ease. He understood their language and customs and he was very good at what he did. A slick customer they used to call him.

But nowadays Vicente never felt much like a slick customer in Miami's tight social circles. He knew he was an outsider trying to fit in, trying not to *feel* like an outsider trying to fit in. And this made him nervous. He never knew if what he said would be right or wrong, it was all a guess for him now. So far he'd proved highly adept at his craft, but the doubt was always there. *What if I say the wrong thing? What if I offend someone?* He constantly questioned himself. Maybe it kept him sharp, the constant self-doubt. He didn't know. All he knew at this moment was that he was once again entering a world he didn't completely understand or enjoy, and it would be an uncomfortable afternoon at best.

In the new post-*Miami Vice* era not every multi-million dollar deal done in Miami involved drugs, at least not directly. Real estate speculation, international trade, banking, the fashion industry – these were becoming as important to 1990's Miami as illegal drugs had been to the city's economy during the 1970's and 1980's. The drugs were still there, but increasingly it was the business of *washing* the money generated from the drugs that helped fuel the economy. As was the flow of petro-dollars from corrupt government officials in South America, or the flight of capital from brethren in the same countries that controlled most of the local and national businesses. It was a new day and a new way that drove Miami's newest expansion, but one constant remained. Regardless of the source of funds, if you were well-liked at this influential level, opportunities could and would open for you almost anywhere.

That was how Enrique had made the transition from criminal and sometimes freedom fighter to respected businessman. Money breeds opportunity, and Enrique was smart with his money, smart enough to gain an entry into a different world. Now the opportunities flowed for him like the vintage Champaigns served at these *soirees*. He was accepted. He was one of *them* now.

"No problem my old friend. I will coach you. All you need to do with this group is try to be charming to the wife of Sandifer. If she likes you, it will not be a problem to learn what you need to know." Enrique's grin was devious but he quickly countered by adding, "This woman could be his daughter, you know? And from time to time she enjoys some *variety* in her relationships."

"How do you know all this crap?" said Vicente, curious but not amused.

"It is my job to know where all the bones are buried, my friend. This helps me to pass into this circle, a *Cubano* in this wilderness of liars and perverts. This woman, she likes a little of everything. Maybe if she even likes you......." Enrique laughed at the thought as he pulled up to the guard station at the subdivision entrance.

"Yes sir, can I help you?" said the guard politely.

"Enrique Ramírez and guest to see Mr. Sandifer."

"Just one moment please," said the guard, taking a second to check a computer printout by his control panel. "Yes, Mr. Ramírez. Please go ahead. Do you know how to get to the residence?"

"Yes. Thanks very much," replied Enrique, and he drove the big car past the upright barrier and down the palm-lined street. "Look at these houses," he said to Vicente almost reverently. "*This*, my friend, is money."

Each street had only three houses. The lots were enormous, even for country club standards and the homes were so large they resembled individual club houses. Mediterranean-style Spanish *villas* were the dominant style, many painted mustard yellow, tan, or white, and their reddish brown ceramic tiled roofs completed the picture. One end of each lot fronted the Intracoastal Waterway, while the other opened out onto sculpted, but understated gardens.

A team of valets patiently awaited the arrival of each guest, and Enrique passed the Cadillac's keys to one of the young *Cubanos* with a twenty dollar bill, adding in Spanish.

"Have the car ready and waiting here in exactly three hours and I'll give you another twenty." The young man smiled and nodded his head, parking the car less than ten feet from the front door. Enrique motioned for them to go in, and they walked up the small flight of steps to the front entrance.

A doorman dressed in a fancy *guayabera* and khaki Armani trousers greeted them in Spanish and ushered them into the portico where an exquisite young blond girl took their names and drink orders. Vicente stood in the entrance hall and tried not to gape openly at the ostentatious scene. Waiters roamed the crowd with appetizers and drinks while a string quartet play serenely in one corner of the great room. A crowd of nearly seventy five stood and conversed comfortably in the huge room, while some had spilled out onto the rear *cabaña* and pool area to chat or admire the water view. *Enrique lives in style*, he thought, *but this is something very different.*

The place reminded Vicente of some of the beachfront casinos in Veradero just prior to the arrival of Fidel, when hoards of eager American tourists gambled their dollars at the tables and drank the night away at clubs like the Copacabana. Those were good days for him, helping to manage Morgenthal's operations at the Riviera Hotel. In the old days he felt like one of the people he now examined coldly from a distance, in control of his life and on top of the world. He shook his head. That was such a long time ago. The stakes in this room were surely comparable for some to the stakes in the gambling business he'd grown up in, he surmised, but with information and business risk taking the place of competition from the New York and Vegas mobs and Batista's corrupt overseer's.

"There! *Amigo*, I see our hosts," said Enrique quietly. "Come, I will introduce you."

The two men walked quickly across the room to a

small crowd gathered near a bay window. Enrique entered the scene as if he was a close relative, breaking into the conversation without hesitation.

"William, so good to see you again." He shook the tall man's hand warmly. "And Jennifer, I hope all is well with you." The old *Cubano* kissed the girl lightly on the cheek and she smiled broadly. "Please allow me to present my very good and old friend Vicente Amarón. Vicente, the Sandifers."

Vicente extended his hand to the well-dressed host but he momentarily ignored the offer.

"So, Enrique, glad you could make it." Sandifer patted Enrique on the shoulder and smiled thinly at Vicente.

Vicente thought he'd seen the same type of look from guys he knew in the Sicilian Mob. They always smiled like that, just before they were about to shoot you.

"And a pleasure to meet you, Mr. Amarón." Sandifer shook his hand limply.

"At you service, *Señor* Sandifer." Vicente smiled, bowing his head slightly.

Sandifer returned his attention to Enrique. "I've been meaning to call you about that financing you're trying to arrange. Mr. Amarón, please forgive me but I must borrow our friend here for a few minutes to discuss something with him." Sandifer looked expectantly at Vicente for a second but quickly continued with, "Good, I hoped you wouldn't mind. Enrique, I have some things for you to go over in my office." The dapper, graying man extended his arm towards an open hallway and Enrique turned to leave.

"Vicente, I will be just a few minutes. Please enjoy yourself. Jennifer is quite the hostess, and I'm sure you will find her to be a very interesting person." Enrique smiled and left before Vicente could react. The pair looked ridiculous walking across the crowded room together, the short, plump Enrique accompanied by the thin, six foot four inch Sandifer. Vicente had little time to react as Jenny, as she liked to be called, seized the opportunity and tugged on his arm to get his attention.

"It's so good to meet an old friend of Enrique's after all this time, " she said with genuine pleasure. "We so seldom have the chance to associate with the Cuban community. It's refreshing to hear a different voice for a change." She was nearly as tall as Vicente, with a flowing mane of light brown hair that cascaded down her back and across her bare shoulders.

Vicente guessed that she must be a second wife or maybe even a third, about twenty-five if he was right. She sipped a rum punch and stared at him intently with her dark brown eyes, a stare that made him feel uncomfortable from the outset.

"*Señora* Sandifer, it is very good to meet you. I have heard many good things of you and you husband."

Vicente concentrated hard on his grammar and pronunciation, trying desperately not to seem as though he'd just arrived from Mariel.

"Please call me Jenny," she said warmly.

"Yes, Jenny. You have a very beautiful home. Have you live here very long?"

"Oh, not really," she said, flashing her large brown eyes. "We bought the place last year just after William and I were married. But we do enjoy it here. Would you like a tour?"

"*Si,* er, yes, I would very much like that." Vicente offered his arm and the shapely young girl obliged with a smile. They walked out to the *cabaña* and he listed attentively while she pointed out various landmarks and important points about the house. The tour continued through the kitchen, where Jenny commented that she liked the space but didn't cook much. Vicente imagined that the real answer was, "not at all."

The pair climbed the coral steps of the huge, arcing stairwell to the second level and continued on towards the guest bedrooms and master suite. The place reminded Vicente of some of the old *villas* he knew as a child growing up outside Havana. *A different time, a very different place*, he thought, smiling to himself.

"And this is the master suite," said Jenny, pointing casually towards the open door.

"Yes, very nice," said Vicente, totally disinterested. "Jenny, may I ask a question from you about you friends the McHenrys?"

"Sure," she smiled. "But come in first. You really must see the bathroom. It's positively gigantic."

She walked ahead of him into a truly large space, a bathroom but more like the size of the spa's Vicente had once visited in Nice. Italian marble floors with a sunken bathtub the size of a small swimming pool, followed by marble columns that separated the shower and bathing area from the dressing room. The view from the dressing area was beautiful, a grand vista of Biscayne Bay with the city of Miami in the background.

"The view from here at night is really wonderful," she said, taking a seat on her velour sofa. "Sometimes I just sit here and stare out at the boats as they go by. I wonder sometimes where they are going."

"Where who is going?"

"The people," she replied wistfully. "Sometime I wonder about the people. Who are they? Are they happy? Do they have families? You know, that kind of thing."

"*Si*, ah, yes. *Señora* Sandifer…"

"Jenny," she corrected.

"Yes, Jenny. When was the last time you talk with you friends?"

Jenny thought for a second and said, "Well, about a week before they went on their trip – you know, they take a sailing trip every year about this time."

"Yes," said Vicente, trying to stay patient. "I have hear about this."

"Well, I had lunch with Madeleine a few weeks ago and she seemed out of sorts. Kind of worried about something. I just thought she was nervous about the trip. You know, she's been getting nervous before they go. But that's been mostly just the last two years." Vicente smiled but said nothing. "I don't think she likes it as much as when she and Donald were younger," the girl continued. "You know how older people can be sometimes – oh, I'm sorry," she gasped, catching herself too late.

"Don't worry," said Vicente with a slight bow. "I do know how can be old people. I am one of them!"

"You? Oh, I don't think you're so old," she smiled.

Vicente knew that smile, and it was not a good sign. That smile, the upward look of her eyes, a flip of her hair over one shoulder. *Not good*, he thought. *I hope this does not go in a bad direction.*

"Thank you for the compliment, *Señora*. So, you are saying about *Señora* McHenry?"

"Yes," Jenny continued. "Anyway, I guess I don't know exactly what was bothering her but I'm pretty sure it wasn't money. You see, they bought that boat brand new from the Fairwinds Marina about two years ago. I think she said it was a Morgan Out Islander 41 Classic. She told me they paid one hundred fifty thousand in cash for it, like it was no big deal. Even for us that would be a good amount of money, but of course, we could do *much* better than that."

Vicente shifted his weight off his bad leg, trying to stay polite through the increasing pain. "Yes, of course. Please go on."

"Well, she did mention one other thing I thought was a bit strange, even for Madeleine. She said that she and Donald had been talking a lot about what they were going to do when they retired, which I thought was odd."

"This was strange to you?"

"Yes. You see, Donald absolutely *loved* the business. I could never see him retiring or even considering handing over partial control of the company to that horrible man, Lloyd Taylor. He's such a toad. He *leers*, you know. He doesn't just stare – he *leers*. He makes me feel like I've rolled around in a trash heap every time I see him. But there are those times when I can't avoid it because William has to discuss business with him. But he gives me the creeps."

Vicente considered this to be very useful information and he was about to excuse himself when the girl continued.

"And he would never give the company to Jo, either."

"Why do you say this?" he asked.

Jenny leaned in slightly and whispered, " Because he didn't trust her. I heard him tell William once that he thought Jo was trying to get him kicked off the Board of Directors. I don't know why exactly, but Donald didn't trust her, either."

Vicente was well pleased with this last tidbit of information and said, "Jenny, thank you for the tour of your beautiful home. It was very nice." He bowed slightly and was about to leave when she interrupted him again.

"Mr. Amarón, I want you know I didn't mean anything by that remark about older people. You see, I like older men. I guess that's obvious, but what I want to say is that I think you're very *interesting*." The girl stood up and approached him slowly, sizing him up with her large brown eyes.

"All that talk about Lloyd makes me feel uncomfortable, even dirty. I feel like I need to wash him off of me, so think I'll take a shower." She turned around and said, "Can you please undue the snap. I can't reach it very easily."

Here it comes, thought Vicente. *Why me?* He said, "Ok, if you wish," and unsnapped the clasp holding her dress together.

The girl reached back and unzipped the light fabric down to her rear, exposing her nude back and waist. Vicente instantly noticed the lack of underclothes, so he immediately backed away from her and turned to leave.

Before he could escape the room, Jenny turned around and allowed the dress to drop to the floor, exposing her exquisite body. Her breasts rose like ripe melons from her chest and her dark brown nipples were hard and erect, like a pair of grapes. She had no tan lines anywhere, and Vicente shook his head, marveling at her beauty.

"Jenny," he said, trying not to gasp, "you are truly a beautiful young woman. Maybe you are the most beautiful woman I have seen in my life." She smiled. "But I am old man, and I must leave you now."

Jenny frowned slightly and sank down on the wide sofa. She pulled her feet up onto the couch and opened he legs, presenting Vicente with a view he hadn't seen in many years. She slid her hand along her left breast and then down between her legs while she looked at him wantonly. It was enough to destroy a weaker man; he took a deep breath and approached her.

"Are you sure?" she said, smiling seductively.

"Jenny, I *must* go." He kissed her hand and she smiled. "Thank you again for the tour. Now I go to find Enrique."

Vicente turned and left the room swiftly, not wanting to look again in her direction. He walked down the long stairway slowly but deliberately, protecting his bad leg which now ached terribly. His only thought was to find Enrique and escape before he did something he would later regret.

Chapter 5

"Eli Rose to see Bill Sexton."

"Is Mr. Sexton expecting you?" asked the secretary.

"No," said Eli, "but he'll see me just the same. We're old friends."

"Fine. I'll tell him you're here." The girl rang Sexton's extension and said, "A Mr. Rose here to see you Mr. Sexton. He says you are old friends. Yes, I see. Yes sir, I'll tell him."

Eli looked expectantly at the girl who glanced up from the receiver.

"It will be just a moment sir. He'll be right with you."

"Thanks." Eli sat on one of the worn out leather chairs in the waiting room, trying to look like he belonged there. Every time he'd visited Bill since his return to Miami, someone invariably recognized him from that one photo the Coast Guard had prematurely released when *El Grupo* had been captured off Key Largo. The years hadn't completely changed his appearance, or at least not enough to grant him the anonymity he preferred.

Bill was just a green beat reporter for the *Herald* when that incident occurred and had been lucky enough to be at the Coast Guard station working on another story when the *Bridgeford* towed the beat up trawler in. He scooped all the major news agencies and finally earned a permanent desk at the newspaper as a result of his story. Eli had come to rely on him as a source of "unofficial" information on various celebrities and important people in Miami during his first stint in the "lost and found" business, and in return, Eli gave Bill first access to the inside stories of the problems he was hired to solve, edited for true identities, of course.

Eli glimpsed his reflection in the mirrored glass of the picture that hung behind the secretary's desk. The image was indistinct, but what he saw made him think that he looked more like his father than ever. In his dreams he still imagined himself to be that young man in the Coast Guard photo, strong and capable. He'd aged quite a bit since then, and it was now obvious. Less hair, a bit grey at the sides. A slight paunch, the recent reward for a few months of easy living. No, he surely didn't feel he resembled the tired, skinny kid that the "Coasties" had marched off the *Bridgeford* in handcuffs almost twenty years ago. *It's not the years, it's the mileage*, he said to himself, but at least his self-confidence was intact.

He was lost in thought just long enough for Bill Sexton to approach unnoticed. "Rose, you old dog. How the hell are you?"

The two men shook hands as Eli stood up. While

not overly tall himself, Eli was much larger than his short, thin-boned friend. But he knew that Bill had a wiry frame and was quite strong for his size, having once watched him wrestle a drunken shrimper with biceps the size of pineapples to the floor at Alabama Jack's. His white short sleeved shirt and baggy black trousers hid his muscular frame very well. Sexton's appearance often led people to underestimate him and assume him to be on the timid side, but a short burst of his strong personality usually corrected that impression.

"Doing well, Bill. I was wondering if you could spare me a few minutes and some answers to a few questions."

"Sure," said Sexton with a smile. "I'll do what I can."

The two men walked down the hallway to the reporter's office, a cramped space with a lone filing cabinet, a chair for occasional guests, and a desk piled impossibly high with papers and a new Canon Typestar 110 electronic typewriter.

"Have a seat," said Bill. "Can I buy you a coffee?"

"No thanks. Listen Bill, I'll cut right to the chase. I'm investigating the disappearance of Donald McHenry and his wife, and I'll bet you're in the know about his activities and finances. I spoke with Phil Rabinowitz over at Metro-Dade PD this morning and he confirmed to me that the daughter, Josephine McHenry, filed a missing persons report almost two weeks ago. She seems genuinely concerned that something's wrong, so what I want to know is, do you have anything else on the family that you can give me that maybe didn't make it into your article?"

"Close the door," said Sexton quietly. He sat back and stroked his thin black hair with his hand. "Eli, you know how these things go. You get a lead, you flesh it out, check your sources, get it approved, run with what ya' got. You know I published only what we could verify." Sexton sat back and looked at Eli calmly as he sipped his now cold coffee.

"I know," said Eli leaning in towards the desk, "but I'm talking about the stuff you've heard, the stuff you suspect and can't print. I need the dirt on this guy, on the whole family. Everything you think might be true but can't put in print."

The trace of a smile crossed the corner of Sexton's mouth as he put down his cup. "Eli, if I tell you this crap, you gotta' promise me to keep it quiet. You can't tell anyone where you heard it otherwise it could be my ass. Got it?"

"Cross my heart," replied Eli, making the gesture with his right hand. "You know we have a deal."

"And you're gonna' owe me one for this."

"Agreed."

Sexton leaned forward a bit and spoke in a hushed but clear voice. "Well, about a year ago I got an anonymous tip over the phone that there was something about McHenry's finances that wasn't kosher. About a week after that call I received a package here with some pretty incriminating materials in it – photos, dates for meetings, copies of ledger entries for large sums of money, that type of stuff. It all seemed disconnected to me, but I started checking the stuff out."

Bill reached down through a stack of papers and

pulled out a legal-sized manila folder with a label on it that read "Ongoing." He handed it across the desk to Eli. "Check out the photos," he said, waiting for Eli to examine them. "They aren't great, but I can tell you for sure that one of the guys is McHenry but I couldn't place other guy."

Eli looked at the photo of two men, one young, one old, sitting on a bench at the 1st Street Pier in South Beach. It had obviously been taken from a long distance using a telephoto lens. McHenry was turned towards the photographer, while his guest was turned slightly at an angle and away from the camera.

"Can't recognize the guy from this picture," said Eli, handing it back to Sexton. "What's the big deal?"

Sexton replaced the folder under the stack of yellowing papers. "The big deal is that while I couldn't ID the guy, a buddy of mine over at the DEA said it looked a lot like Paco Gutiérrez." Sexton waited for Eli to ask the obvious question and when he didn't, he continued.

"The DEA suspects Francisco "Paco" Gutiérrez is the guy overseeing narcotics distribution in Miami for Pablo Escobar, the current head of the Medellín Cartel."

That got Eli's attention. "So the million dollar question is, why are these two guys having a nice chat on a sunny afternoon?"

"Exactly," replied Sexton. "Why would these guys even know each other in the first place? That started me digging." Sexton reached into another pile of papers and pulled out some hand written notes he'd compiled. He glanced at them and continued. "So then I took a long look at the ledger entries, the dates and times. I can't prove it, but I think the dates and times correspond to meetings like the one photographed at 1st Street Pier, and the ledger entries represent payments."

He handed the notes to Eli. "But these dates – they go back more than two years. And the ledger entries – if these are dollar amounts, they're huge." Eli was fascinated but still unclear where Bill was going with the conversation.

"Right," said Bill with grin. "I had an accountant friend at First National Bank do a quick review of McHenry-Taylor's books for me and like Gomer Pyle used to say – "Surprise, surprise." The same amounts were deposited to the McHenry-Taylor corporate account one week after each of the dates on the list."

Eli leaned back and rubbed his chin. "So you think McHenry is taking payola from the cartels? I don't get it."

"Here's where it gets interesting," smiled Sexton, as if it already wasn't so. "I did some more digging around the social scene down in Bal Harbour. Seems like one of the McHenrys has a little coke problem." Before Eli could ask, Bill said, "Yep, I think it's the daughter, Josephine."

No shit, Eli thought to himself. *Didn't see that one coming, but no surprise. I must be slipping.*

"So here's my theory," Bill continued. "But remember, I can't prove any of this. The daughter has herself a little cocaine "Jones" and someone in the local distribution network clues Paco in that they have a rich client with connections. Paco get's a meeting with McHenry and blackmails him into laundering cartel money through his business. It's perfect, really.

McHenry-Taylor is a private company, so they don't have to worry about filing public financial reports. They can bury the money in legitimate transactions and funnel it back to the cartels through offshore bank accounts in McHenry-Taylor's name. McHenry gets to keep his dirty laundry a secret, skims a commission for himself and the company, and the cartels get a clean source of funds." Bill sat back and took another sip of his now rancid coffee, grimacing at the taste. He put the cup on the window sill.

"Well, that would definitely explain a lot of things," said Eli slowly. "Something like that would get pretty unhealthy after awhile. I'd want to disappear if I was Donald McHenry. Maybe hop a boat for the farthest tropical island I could find where nobody knew me and no one could find me." He thought about it silently for a second.

"Yeah, that sounds like a good plan to me."

Sexton stood up and motioned for Eli to open the door. "Eli, once again, I'm only guessing here. I can't prove any of this and I could be dead wrong about all of it." He paused for a second. "But I don't think so. I think this guy McHenry is dirty. I think the whole family is dirty, and that's what's going on here. Just don't quote me on any of it."

Eli got up and shook Bill's hand. "Don't worry, buddy. I won't tip anyone off." He turned to leave and added, "But I can't guarantee I won't be making some waves pretty soon."

Sexton held onto his hand for a moment, causing Eli to stop and look at him. "Eli, remember our deal. You owe me, and I want an exclusive on this one. No bullshit, you give me everything when you've wrapped this one up. I don't want to be reading about this in the *Wall Street Journal*."

Eli smiled and paused in the doorway. "Don't worry, Bill. I promise. Once I get to the bottom of this you'll be the first to know."

§

"Enrique, where the hell have you been?" said Vicente, exasperated.

His friend shot back a puzzled look but put his arm around Vicente and directed him out towards the pool. "Come with me. I have some things to tell you."

The two men walked slowly through the crowd, emerging onto the coral stone pool deck. They found a place to talk near the stone railing that separated the pool area from the walkway to the boat dock.

"*Amigo*," Enrique began, "did you have some type of problem? Why are you so angry?"

Vicente was incensed but controlled himself, not wanting to offend his old *compadre*. "You left me alone with that girl. Do you know what she try to do?"

Enrique burst out laughing but immediately tried to stifle himself. "So, you were introduced to the charms of the beautiful Mrs. Sandifer?" He laughed again and said, "I suppose it was not fair of me to do that to you."

"And you know she do this type of thing?" whispered Vicente.

"Oh, yes. Everyone knows this. She likes the older men. Just look at who she has married."

"And the husband, *he* know of this?"

Enrique chuckled. "Yes, he knows, my friend. And he tolerates it. The rumor is that the guy even likes to watch from a hidden place while the wife does what she does best. I think maybe they are a very good match."

"My God, what crazy shit," whispered Vicente.

"Well, my old friend, you know the saying – there is someone for everyone. Now, do you want to know what I found out or do you want to talk more about this woman?"

Vicente leaned back against the railing and folded his arms. "Ok, *amigo*, tell me what you know."

Enrique leaned against the railing next to Vicente and fingered his watch nervously. "You must tell no one about how you know this, not even Eli, understand?" Vicente stared at his friend in a questioning manner but nodded slightly in agreement. "Very good. I talked with Sandifer about our business together and managed to direct the conversation to the subject of our competitors, including McHenry-Taylor. Sandifer tells me that there is a rumor that McHenry has some personal trouble in his family that has carried over into the business. His partner, Lloyd Taylor was about to convene a meeting of the Board of Directors and the thought is that maybe he had convinced them to remove Donald from his position as CEO. Maybe this is why the guy disappears." Enrique seemed very satisfied with himself, and folded his arms to copy Vicente's pose.

"*Si, amigo*, this is very important to know," said Vicente with a smile. "This is very important."

"Good, I am happy to be of service," said Enrique, patting Vicente on the back. "Especially now that you owe me dinner."

"What?" said Vicente in mock protest. "This no was part of the deal."

"Sorry old friend, but that is my price. You know, those damn doctors have me on such a restricted diet that sometimes I need to have some real food."

"So what you are thinking?"

Enrique smiled. "We go to the Versailles to eat some good Cuban food. And please do not tell me I cannot have what I want."

Vicente gave his old friend a hug and the two men started back through the crowd towards the door. "Don't worry, *amigo*. I no want to be the food police. You can have whatever you want."

Chapter 6

"Rita, has Vicente called in yet?" Eli wanted to know what Vicente had discovered in Bal Harbour. After his visit with Bill Sexton, he was certain that the cocaine connection was the key to the McHenrys disappearance. He needed Vicente to run down any leads on Gutiérrez and find out what he knew.

"Yes. He and Enrique Ramírez stopped at the Versailles for a late lunch and he's on his way back to the office."

"Tell him to wait for me. I should be there in half an hour."

Eli drove his old GTO through the Brickell Avenue traffic as quickly as he dared, but not at the breakneck speed of his youth. The old car had seen better days, and its inefficient drum brakes couldn't handle the sudden stops required of that stretch of lights across from Bayfront Park. *One of these days I'll get this thing fixed*, he thought. But that would have to wait until after the McHenry disappearance had been resolved, one way or the other.

He arrived at the Lincoln Center tower and impatiently rode the elevator up to the 21st floor. "Is Vicente in his office?" Eli quizzed Rita as he burst through the door.

"Yes," she replied without looking up from her new Dell computer.

He knocked on the door but entered before Vicente could answer.

"Vicente, we need to talk."

"*Si, amigo.* I know. I have many thing to tell you." He had his feet propped up on the desk and had been scribbling notes on a small pad.

"Ok, then," said Eli as he sat down opposite his friend. "You first."

Vicente reached for his note pad before he continued. "You know Eli, I no like to do this type of work. Sometime maybe is Ok but these type of people I no like."

"I understand, Vicente, but you're the guy who can pull it off. I'm not "distinguished looking" enough to fit in."

The old man frowned and looked at his notes. "Ok, I only want to tell you this but I accept that the job is for me. Just not too many times. The people are very strange." He paused to emphasize his distaste for the whole affair.

"So, Eli, Enrique and I, we go to a party in Bal Harbour to meet some of these very important people. These people, they are friends to the man Donald McHenry and his wife. The big message we have from this people is that McHenry had much money trouble and maybe he is lose his position in the company very soon." He flipped to the next page in the pad.

"His partner, Lloyd Taylor want to make it very difficult for Donald to stay as CEO, so the man was think about his future a lot. I also hear from a friend of the wife Madeleine that she no was happy to have her usual vacation this year and that they have a lot of money. They buy the new boat for cash, one hundred fifty thousand dollars." Vicente tossed the pad on the desk and smiled.

"This people the McHenrys no are good people I think. Maybe the girl, she know or does not know. What do you think?"

"I think that's very good information." Eli picked up the note pad for a second and then replaced it on the desk. "I think that what I learned is very consistent with what you just told me, just maybe with another layer of detail."

Eli walked over to the door and said to Rita, "No calls unless it's Jo McHenry." Rita just waved, still transfixed on the new computer.

"I went over to see Bill Sexton at the *Herald* and he had quite a story to tell. He can't prove much of what he suspects, but it looks like our employer has herself a little cocaine habit. A lowlife named Paco Gutiérrez picked up on it and was blackmailing the old man into laundering cartel money through his company to keep it all quiet. Jo must know more about this than she's telling us; I'll have a talk with her while we're in the Bahamas."

"The Bahamas?"

Eli smiled. "Yes, I'm traveling again. Jo insisted that she wasn't going to let us just do our jobs and report back to her. She's going to come along and "assist" in the investigation. I could have dumped her on you, but I figured you'd be pretty mad if I did that."

Vicente shook his head and said, "Thank you for no give this lady to me. I have much to do and no have time to be her *caudillo*."

Eli pulled a map from his pocket and unfolded it on the desk. "So let me show you the plan, in case something goes wrong and I need some help. Tomorrow we'll take the Bahamasair flight to Nassau and check in at the Graycliff. I already have a meeting set up with Leslie Robertson at the RBDF. I think you know him." Vicente nodded in the affirmative.

"I've reserved a boat for Friday and I plan to sail to Andros Town and sort of blend in with the sailing crowd so we can ask some questions without getting the local's curiosity up. If I have any leads after that I'll call you again from Nassau, probably next Tuesday. If you don't hear from me then call Leslie and have him come looking for us."

"Ok, Eli. I will do this."

"That's not everything, Vicente. I need you to set up a meeting with Lloyd Taylor and find out what he knows about McHenry and his finances. I think he may have been the one to tip off the government. Maybe he's trying to use the situation to leverage McHenry out of the company. Anyway, let's see if he's as righteous as he seems or if he's in on this monkey business. And find a way to contact this guy Paco Gutiérrez. Play up the angle that you have old friends down south that will help him out if he lets you in on things. I'm sure you can come up with a good story. We probably need to get rid of this guy to protect the girl, but let's first see what he can tell us about the old man and their deal."

Vicente paused and stared intently at Eli for a moment.

"Eli, you know this is very dangerous to do this thing, *si*? You no will be easy to find if there is a problem, and I think this asshole Gutiérrez is a very bad guy. If I start this with him you know where it will end, understand?"

"Yes, I know. But I think it's the only way we're going to get to the bottom of this deal. Otherwise we'll be scraping along the edges for a year with nothing much to go on. Trust me on this one, old friend."

"*Si*, I trust you," said Vicente with a sly smile. "We will do this like the old days, I think. Is Ok if I ask for some help from the old friends?"

Eli knew what he meant and didn't like it, but since Vicente would be on his own he could hardly object.

"Sure, but just keep their involvement to a minimum. Ok, I need to get a few things ready before tomorrow. Give my travel details and Leslie's phone number to Rita so she can keep tabs on me. Same for you, too. Don't make any serious moves without telling her."

Eli stood and embraced his friend. "If everything goes right I'll have some answers in a week or so and we can close this one up. After that we'll close up for awhile and take a nice, peaceful vacation someplace."

"This sound very good to me. Go with God my friend."

Eli went to his desk and pulled out the Beretta and his extra clips. He hoped he wouldn't need it, but caution was the best policy when cruising the Bahamas, and the gun would definitely be of service in a tight situation. He stopped by Rita's desk before he left the office and gave her a kiss on the cheek.

"Mind the office while I'm away and be sure to look after the old man," he said quietly. "I'll be away for about a week but I may call in next Tuesday. Vicente's got all the details. Please make sure to keep tabs on him for me. If he gets into trouble he's gonna' need your help."

"Don't worry, I'll watch out for him," she replied with a note of concern in her voice.

He smiled and left, heading home to pack his things for the task that lay ahead.

§

The front doorbell rang loudly and the sound bounced around off the tile floors like an echo. The house looked much the same from a distance, but closer inspection showed it was in a state of disrepair. Entropy and a lack of funds had taken the once exotic entrance from compelling to almost tragic in the space of twenty years. That was how Vicente felt about himself as well. *I have really gone downhill*, he thought. *Twenty years ago I was so much more than I am now. Where did the time go?* He discarded the thought as the old wooden door opened.

"Vicente, old friend! How are you?" Julio immediately embraced his old friend warmly and smiled broadly. "It has been a very long time. Almost twenty years, no? Please come in."

The furnishings had changed a bit but Vicente immediately felt comfortable in the old house. "Please sit. Can I get you a drink?"

"No thanks. So, Julio, how have you been?" Vicente was relieved to be able to speak Spanish with his old compatriot. At least Julio was still willing to speak it at this point.

Julio sat on the sofa next to Vicente and rubbed his ample belly while pointing to the top of his bald head. "As you can see, I am bigger than I was when we last saw each other and I have no hair, but otherwise I am Ok. Money is another thing, but basically I am Ok. And you are looking very well, *amigo*. What are you doing these days?"

"I am working again with Eli. We have a new office on Brickell Avenue. You should come by for a visit some time."

"Ah, yes. I heard Eli was back in Miami. So, old friend, I maybe can guess you are not here on a social call. What is it that I can do for you?" Julio sat back and stared hard at Vicente in the way he did when they were both in *El Grupo*.

"I need some help to contact a guy," said Vicente hesitantly. "This guy - he is really bad, but I need to get inside his organization. Maybe you can help?" Julio replied, "Tell me who is the guy and then I will tell you if I can help."

"The guy is called Paco Gutiérrez."

Julio's eyes widened as the name cleared Vicente's lips. He stood up and put his hands in his pockets and walked over to look out his sliding glass door at his patio. He shook his head and said, "Do you know who is this guy? When you said that he is a bad guy, you have no idea how bad he really is. I cannot help you."

Vicente approached his fat friend, palms open. "I know who is this guy, but I need to meet him. Can't you even arrange for this, for your old friend?"

"Let me tell you a story," replied Julio. "Your friend, Paco Gutiérrez, he is maybe the most dangerous man in Miami. You know he is connected to the Medellín Cartel? He has many soldiers working for him and they kill anyone who gets too close. No matter if they are Anglo or *Cubano*, you ask too many questions and you disappear. Then maybe they find you cut into little pieces and floating in the Miami River like fish food. Trust me old friend, you do not want to meet this guy."

"So you know how to contact him?"

Julio sighed audibly and shook his head. "I know some people who know some people. And tell me, why are you so interested in ending your life? After all of our struggles together and everything we have done, to throw it away in this manner - I don't understand."

"Julio, I am on a job. This guy Gutiérrez has information that will help me with a very important case, and so I must talk with him. Will you help me or not?"

"I need a drink." Julio exited the room and Vicente could hear him in the kitchen grumbling under his breath while he poured himself a rum on ice. He returned and gulped the drink, nearly coughing from the intensity of the alcohol.

"I don't drink very much these days," he mused. "My doctor say I must cut back, that it's not good for my liver. Bah - what does he know?" Julio downed the glass and exhaled mightily. "So you want to meet this shit Gutiérrez? If you believe you must do this, I can arrange a meeting."

Vicente smiled and patted his friend on the shoulder. "I knew all along that you could do this. So when can we have the meeting?"

Julio sighed again. He never could resist a sincere request from Vicente, especially after their long shared history of struggle against the Cuban government.

"Ok, *amigo*. We can use our past life to get you into this guy's inner circle. But once you are there I cannot help you. Understand?" Vicente nodded.

"Good. So I will tell this friend of a friend that I know a guy with good connections in Pinar del Rio, someone who has a good dialogue with the generals in Cuba and who can maybe help to facilitate the transit of materials from Cuba to Miami. In this way, you do not have to use a cover. You can be who you are, and who knows? Maybe you will survive for a few days." Julio put his drink on the coffee table and then grabbed his friend by both shoulders.

"But I will tell you again, Vicente. The old team is not active these days, so we cannot help you if you get into trouble. You will be only a guy that was presented to me, and I am passing you along. That's all."

Vicente nodded again and said, "I understand my friend. I don't want to put you at risk. This is my problem if things don't go well."

"Ok. Let me make the contact and I will call you. You have a business card?"

Vicente reached into his shirt pocket and produced a slightly creased card for Brickell Avenue Associates.

"If I am not there you can leave a message with the girl."

Julio inspected the number, holding the card at a distance with his outstretched arm.

"My eyes are not so good anymore old friend. Look at what we have come to! Ah, Ok, I see it. Yes, I will call you when I have the day, time, and place arranged."

"Thank you," said Vicente, turning to leave. He walked to the door and Julio stopped him with a small tug at his arm.

Julio switched to English to ask Vicente one final question.

"Vicente, whatever happened to that son of a bitch Robert Jasper? Do you know anything about him? I would still like to kill him for what he did to us back there, when the Coast Guard got us."

"No," Vicente replied in English.. "I no see him again. But I think maybe he is with the Devil in Hell. Thanks very much, Julio. We speak soon."

The old man smiled and walked out. He realized it was better to avoid telling Julio what really happened to Jasper so he could keep him cooperative and focused on the job at hand.

Vicente decided to stop at Monty's Bayshore in Coconut Grove for a quick beer and to call Rita. He needed to try and get a meeting with Lloyd Taylor as soon as possible and needed Rita to work her magic. She seemed to be able to set up meetings with everyone from important business men to local politicians with ease. He didn't know how she did it, but he needed her talents one more time.

"Rita, I am on pay phone at Monty's. Tell me if he has time today. I wait at this number until you call me back."

"Sure, Ok. Hang on and I'll let ya' know." Vicente sat by the phone and stared out at the growing crowd, approaching for yet another Happy Hour by Sailboat Bay. He sipped his beer slowly, careful not to finish too soon, and stared down the two guys who looked like they wanted to make a call. They seemed to get the message without a word having been exchanged. After what seemed to him like an eternity, the telephone rang and Vicente grabbed the receiver immediately.

"Rita, is you?"

"Yeah, is me," she said, mocking his accent. "Do ya' wanna' know what I have or not?"

"*Si*, please go ahead."

"So Lloyd Taylor is booked up all day, but his secretary says he will see you if you want to meet him for a drink at The Forge at seven. He has a business dinner there with some clients at eight, so that's your window."

"Ok, very good. Please to tell his secretary I meet him there at seven. *Gracias*, Rita."

"You're welcome old man. Don't screw this up or Eli will kill you."

She hung up and Vicente began to sweat. He had just enough time to get back to his place in Little Havana, shower and change into some evening clothes so he could present his best impression to Taylor. *I will get there at six thirty and have a big rum before the guy gets there*, he thought.

He arrived at the old restaurant at six fifteen and the gave the valet twenty dollars when he handed him the key to the old Corvette.

"Keep it safe and clean and I give you twenty more when I am done," he said to the valet in English. Vicente couldn't tell whether he was a Salvadoran or a Honduran, certainly from one of those places. The kid was skinny, probably barely able to make ends meet. Vicente saw himself reflected in the kid's expectant eyes: young, naive, ready to tackle anything for a chance to get ahead. He'd been the same way when he was that age, and that's how he'd managed to climb into Batista's inner circle before working for Morgenthal.

The kid replied, "*Si, Señor*, no problem," and quickly moved the old machine to the restaurant's valet lot. Vicente shook his head and smiled, wondering if this kid was destined for a similar future.

Another valet welcomed him in by opening the large door and Vicente was back in the place he'd known in better times. Not a large room by any means, but an ornately decorated space with red and gold trim in abundance. It was a favorite of the Hollywood elite in its heyday during the 1960's, and Vicente often accompanied Morgenthal there when he met with visiting members of the New York crime families. The place brought back pleasant memories for him and helped him to relax a bit. A stiff drink would help him even more.

"Rum and soda," he said to the bartender as he took a seat.

Vicente scanned the room and saw no sign of Lloyd Taylor, which was what he expected. *A man with that much money is never early and rarely on time unless he really wants to be,* he thought. He sipped his drink and reviewed his planned dialogue with Taylor. It would go something like:

1) *I am with the investigative team hired by Josephine McHenry to locate her parents.*

2) *In order for our investigation to be successful I must ask you a few questions.*

3) *What can you tell me about Donald McHenry's finances? Was he in any trouble?*

That should be enough to get things started, he thought. He hoped he would be able to get the guy talking about his partner and boss in a relaxed setting away from the rigid confines of his office. *Maybe after a couple of drinks he will loosen up?* He didn't know but hoped for the best.

At precisely seven in the evening a small entourage entered the restaurant and at the rear of the group was Lloyd Taylor. Vicente had seen his photo but had not met him in person. Taylor was taller and appeared to be in better physical condition than Vicente. His bespoke Savile Row suit fit him like a light gray glove, and the unscuffed, highly polished black Bally shoes and matching belt suggested a fastidiousness with his public image. *This guy is rich,* thought Vicente. *Very rich.* And it was clear that he spent his money on what he considered to be the finer things in life.

Taylor motioned for his bodyguards to have a seat at the back of the bar and then walked directly up to Vicente and said, "You must be Mr. Amarón. My name is Lloyd Taylor. Mind if I sit down?"

"Is a pleasure sir. Yes, please have a seat." Vicente motioned for him to sit with his back towards the door. It was an old habit that died hard, but he always wanted to have a view of the door in case something unexpected occurred.

"Thank you for agree to meet me on short notice."

"Certainly," said Taylor. "It was no problem since I was going to be here anyway. Bartender - Glenlivet on the rocks please." The bartender nodded and Taylor returned his attention to Vicente.

"So, you are the man Jo McHenry hired to find her parents. Tell me about yourself. How long have you been doing this type of work?"

Vicente was taken by surprise by his question, which was uncommon in his experience. Usually it was he who had the upper hand in such situations, but now Taylor was asking the questions and Vicente was forced to respond. *I am getting too old for this,* he thought.

"Our company is doing this type of work almost twenty year," Vicente replied, hoping Taylor wouldn't check. "We have much experience with this type of thing and many satisfied clients."

"Good. Glad to hear that," answered Taylor. He smiled as the bartender placed his drink on the bar and quickly grabbed the glass. "Cheers," he said. "Let's hope your efforts are successful very soon." The two men clinked glasses and Taylor took a deep sip of his scotch.

"I presume you want to ask me some questions about Donald. I will of course help you any way I can."

The man's hands were steady as a rock, as was the gaze from his steely blue eyes. Vicente could see that

Taylor was a direct, no nonsense type, so he proceeded directly to the matter at hand.

"Mr. Taylor, there is some rumor about the financial affairs of Mr. McHenry, specifically about the source of his personal finance and the money he was invest into the company. Can you help me to understand the situation?"

Taylor took another deep drink and drained the glass. "Another, please," he said the bartender.

"For two years now the company has been struggling to get by. The economy is down and high-end goods are not selling like they were a few years ago. I had been pushing Donald to alter our product line to include more moderately priced clothing, but he insisted that we maintain ourselves at the upper end. He believed very strongly that high-end fashions would regain their luster and we'd be foolish to change our brand image now that times were difficult."

Taylor sat back in his chair and again drank deeply from his new glass.

"More than a year ago I noticed something odd. It started out as a simple accounting error, or that's what I thought. Then it became a regular event, these monthly deposits to the company's accounts. When I questioned Donald about it he said some other investments had paid out and he'd cleared it with the Board to take additional equity in the company in exchange for his infusion of capital. I was suspicious of where the money was coming from, but I could not get him to tell me any more than that. In addition, he seemed to be doing better personally as well. That's all I know."

Vicente nodded his approval but could tell that

Taylor was not telling him the truth, or at least not everything. Although the words were spoken calmly, they were hollow, completely free of emotion.

"Sir, so you no make this a problem for McHenry with the Directors? My information say that you think his activity was to make very risky the future of you company. That maybe what he was doing no was legal."

Taylor sighed and rubbed his hand through his thin graying hair.

"Look, this was pretty clear. Donald wouldn't tell me where the funds were coming from and I couldn't take the chance that the source was from something less than legal, if you understand what I'm saying. I mean, look what happen to De Lorean. I couldn't take that risk because it could bring down the entire company. So I scheduled a Board meeting to review the situation while Donald and Madeleine were on their annual sailing trip. I felt like we could get through it and present Donald with some "options" when he returned."

"What type of "options" do you mean?"

"I wanted him either to step down as CEO or sell his interest in the company and retain the title in name only. I thought that a little pressure applied in the right places might "convince" him."

Vicente felt like that part of the story rang true, and it was consistent with what he'd heard from Eli and his other sources up to this point.

"So why you no have the meeting?"

Taylor smiled and tossed down the rest of his drink. He stared directly into Vicente's eyes, seemingly searching for how much he felt he could safely reveal.

"Well, Jo McHenry "persuaded" me to reconsider. She said she would get to the bottom of the situation when her father returned. She only wanted me to wait two more weeks before I called the meeting. It sounded reasonable, so I've decided to wait a bit longer and see what happens. But as we can see, something clearly isn't right and she hasn't been able to find Donald and Madeleine. But then, that's why you're here."

"Yes, that is why I am here. You say that the girl "persuade" you not to call the meeting now. What is this exactly? What did she tell you?"

The restaurant door opened at that moment and a group of very well-dressed men entered with some extremely attractive and much younger women at their sides. "Ah, my guests have arrived," said Taylor standing up.

"I'm afraid I must go now. It was a pleasure to meet you Mr. Amarón and I hope I was able to help with your investigation. Good luck."

"Yes, sir," replied Vicente rising and shaking his hand. "Thank you for you time."

As Taylor started to leave Vicente held tight to his hand, squeezing down hard. He'd used the same tactics to get the attention of certain mobsters in the old days. It was an outwardly subtle, yet very noticeable way to hold one's attention.

"One more thing, sir. So you say the girl "persuade" you. Please tell me how."

Taylor tried to pull his hand away suddenly but Vicente's vice-like grip held fast. He grimaced but tried not to show his discomfort to his guests, who had noticed him at the bar and waved to him from their table.

"Fine, I'll tell you. Now let go."

Vicente eased his grip and Taylor quickly withdrew his hand.

"You've met Jo, so you know she has some very obvious "assets" that she uses to her advantage from time to time. I've had the good fortune of getting to know her in a more "personal" way of late and as you know, she can be quite charming when she wants to be. Do I need to be more specific, or will that do?"

"That is very good information. Thank you very much for you time, *Señor* Taylor."

Vicente stepped aside and Taylor brushed past him in a cloud of cologne. Vicente thought he should have asked him what brand he used because it smelled elegant. He smiled to himself and sat down to finish his drink. *So there is much more to this girl than she shows on the surface,* he thought. *She is playing a very serious game and who knows what else she is hiding?*

The bartender interrupted his train of thought and asked, "Sir, will you be joining us for dinner?"

Vicente contemplated the thought for a second and then felt a burst of energy. "*Si*, I think I will stay. I am feel pretty good tonight. Maybe you can bring to me a steak here?" He handed the bartender a twenty and the guy smiled.

"Certainly, sir. Whatever you like."

The old man looked across the bar at his reflection in the small mirrored wall and was pleased. He looked good tonight, almost like in the old days. And he'd extracted a critical piece of information from Taylor about the girl, something Eli didn't know. *I will call Eli tonight*, he said to himself. *Then I will celebrate like it was the old days.*

Chapter 7

I'm gonna' kill that girl, Eli thought as he waited impatiently at the Bahamasair air ticket counter. He hated Miami International even on the best of days, but they could not afford to miss this flight as the other flights were sold out and the crowd behind him was nearly ready to riot.

"Can ya' believe this shit?" said the young guy behind him. Eli turned to look at the guy, a short but thin rich kid dressed in his Gucci loafers and wearing his Wayfarers indoors to make himself look "cool." His very annoyed girlfriend hung on his arm and smacked her gum, firing off disgusted looks at anyone who made eye contact.

"They cancel one flight and the whole damn world shows up early so they can try to get on this one."

"Yes, pretty inconvenient," replied Eli curtly.

"Yeah, right. Someone oughta' do somethin'," said the kid.

That got Eli's attention. "Really? What would you suggest?"

The kid, apparently feeling an endorsement of his

indignation turned to his girl and said, "Wait here, honey. I'm gonna' have a word with that bitch at the desk."

He proceeded to push his way to the front of the line and the Bahamasair desk, where his agitated hand gestures and waves back towards the crowd were met with blank stares. His insistence quickly produced a burly security guard and then another. Not sensing what was about to happen, the guy slammed his fist down in front of the now shocked desk assistant and that was it. The security guards grabbed the guy and began dragging him out to the breezeway, where three uniformed Miami Dade police officers were happy to greet him. His girlfriend grabbed her bag and jumped out of line to follow him, yelling at the cops while he protested as they half-carried him out the automatic doors.

The distraction was good for Eli because it slowed the check-in for the flight and allowed more time for his painfully late boss to arrive.

"Sorry," she said, strolling up to him in a casual fashion. "I had some trouble finding everything I needed this morning. Your list was so specific: a broad-brimmed hat, suntan lotion, bathing suits, dressy casual evening wear. I can't just throw all that stuff together, you know."

Eli had learned well from his previous employers to bite his tongue and say nothing when he was angry with their behavior.

"Well, good morning to you, too. Sorry if I made things difficult for you."

Jo stared at him, immediately reading the sarcasm

in his voice.

"Yes. Well, I'm here and that's what counts."

She was stunning as usual, dressed in tight white shorts and a multicolored blouse that was opened to the top of her cleavage. She wore a pair of dressy white open-toed sandals and carried her wide-brimmed white hat with her. Eli couldn't see her eyes through the dark Persol sunglasses but he guessed they were a bit bloodshot from a night of partying.

"So, you look tired this morning. Had a late night last night? Need a cup of coffee?"

She pulled off her glasses and glared at him, clear-eyed as usual. "It was a fantastic party. Too bad you couldn't be there."

"Having my beauty sleep," he replied. "Besides, I had a few last minute details to work through before we left. Anyway, I didn't know I was invited."

"You weren't."

"Next," said the girl at the desk. Eli and Jo stepped up and Eli presented their tickets. "Passports, please," she said as she logged the tickets into the computer. Jo reached into her small white and gold Gucci bag and shoved the document at Eli. He handed both over to the girl and just smiled.

"So, Mr. Rose, Ms. McHenry, you will be in 2A and 2B. Your bags are checked to Nassau and we'll be leaving from gate twenty three, A concourse. Have a nice flight."

"Thanks," said Eli. He held the passports and tickets while they exited the line. "Ok, here you go. Do you have a seat preference?"

"Not really," she said. "I plan on sleeping. It's only

an hour or so anyway, isn't it?"

"About fifty five minutes. Let's go wait at the gate."

Eli led the way through security and they walked down to the departure gate. The old fabric chairs were worn through and torn in various spots, so Jo carefully positioned herself on the edge of the best looking seat.

"So, where are we staying?" she said with little interest.

"A place called the Graycliff. I've stayed there several times when visiting friends. I think you'll like it."

Jo sniffed and grabbed a tissue from her purse. "I normally stay on the boat when we go to the Bahamas," she answered, dabbing at her nose.

"Have a cold?" Eli asked suspiciously. He suspected a "coke-induced" nasal problem.

"No, just the temperature change. They keep it like an icebox in here."

Eli just smiled but was contemplating the days upcoming events. After they checked into the hotel he'd take a taxi out to the RBDF headquarters for his meeting with Leslie Robertson. Then he'd go check on the boat at the marina to be sure everything was ready for the trip. It would take about twelve hours to get to Andros Town, so he'd need to get to sleep pretty early.

After a brief delay they boarded the flight and settled into their first class seats. The plane was one of Bahamasair's new 737's, so they had a more comfortable cabin for the brief hop over to Nassau. Jo immediately dozed off as the plane departed Miami, still wearing her sunglasses while Eli stared out the window at the water, looking at the wave patterns that flowed over the Great Bahama Bank.

The sun was out and the water looked crystal clear from above, and Eli hoped the weather stayed stable during the trip. At this time of year anything can happen, and hurricanes can quickly spring up almost out of nowhere in this part of the Caribbean. Just as quickly as they'd reached cruising altitude, Eli felt the plane begin to descend towards Nassau. Jo was roused by the stewardess on the intercom.

"Please return your seatbacks and tray tables to their upright and locked positions," she said in her sing-song Bahamian accent. "On behalf of the flight crew I want to thank you for flying Bahamasair, and have a pleasant stay."

Jo straightened herself up and pulled a mirror out of her purse. "How do I look," she said, staring at Eli."

"Like a million bucks."

"That's not what I meant. Do I look presentable enough to meet your friend at the Defense Force?"

Eli's heart sank. He'd hoped she would be occupied unpacking or getting herself ready for the trip the next day, leaving him to meet Leslie alone. But that hope vanished immediately and he knew that protesting would only result in a rebuke and a lecture.

"Sure, you look great," he sighed.

They managed to slip through immigration like the rest of the tourists but it was customs that Eli feared. He'd stuffed the Beretta and the loaded clips into his bag, knowing that Bahamasair did not screen their baggage like the US airlines, but now he had to hope they wouldn't be stopped for a random check. Jo had her hat and sunglasses on and she truly did look like a million bucks, so Eli had her move forward with her bag first.

"Miss, can you step over here please?" said a well-appointed guard. "Just a random check. Sorry to inconvenience you." He motioned for Jo to put her bag on a nearby table while the guard immediately in front of Eli said, "You can wait for her over there, sir."

"Thanks," Eli replied. He looked over at the distressed girl and just shrugged his shoulders. It was his good fortune not to be the one that was stopped and searched, as he would have had to call Leslie to get him out of trouble. Now he'd have his weapon of choice for the duration of the trip.

Jo stood by with her hands on her hips while the customs agents looked through her personal affects. "Thanks, Miss. You can go." Jo obviously thought better of saying anything so she just re-packed her bag quickly and joined Eli by the exit to the terminal.

"Are you done fooling around?" Eli chided.

"Better watch out, buster. I'm really mad right now, and you won't like me when I'm mad."

The girl's face was flushed red and even though he couldn't see her eyes, Eli knew she would have bored a hole right through him if she could.

"Sorry. Just pulling your leg. Let's get a taxi and go check in at the hotel." He picked up her bag and flagged down the first free taxi at the stand. "Graycliff Hotel, if you please."

"Yeah, soulja'," replied the young driver, smiling. He loaded the bags into his trunk and opened the door for Jo. "In ya' go sweet pie."

Jo looked at Eli quizzically and he just smiled. "Bahamians use a dialect that is unique to the islands, and it can be pretty colorful," he whispered.

"So, ya' goin' ta' Graycliff. You is American?"

"Yes," said Eli.

"Ah, is good. And you is?"

"I'm Eli. This is Jo. And you is?" Eli didn't go too far down the road using local slang, but he used some for effect, especially to put people at ease.

The young guy smiled into the rear-view mirror, prominently displaying two gold teeth. "I is Carlton. Carlton Lawson. Ya' no Conchy Joe, eh general?"

"What did he just call you?" said Jo, perplexed.

"He just asked if I was a Bahamian," said Eli.

"Ya' right, man. Very good. Dis' ma' taxi an I be at ya' service." Carlton looked back and tipped his black beret. "Is ya' woman ah ya' sweethart?" he said to Eli.

"Neither one. She's my boss."

"Ah, Lord. Ya' lucky man, have a boss like dat.' She gotta' boonggy dat' world class, man."

Carlton laughed and Eli just shook his head. "In case you're wondering," he said to Jo, "he said you have a world class rear." Jo looked aghast and Carlton just laughed. Eli shrugged and smiled.

"I could have guessed it was something like that," she said. "I'll take it as a compliment, Mr. Carlton," she said leaning forward. He smiled and nodded his head.

They arrived at the hotel in a few minutes and Carlton delivered the bags to the bellman. "Deez' ma' friends, boy. Don' mess up dey stuff or ah come back an muggage you up real fine. Ya' got it?" The bellman grunted but carefully carried the bags into the lobby.

"Here ya' go, Carlton," said Eli, handing him twenty dollars. "Definitely worth the trip."

"Ya' alright, general." Carlton shook his hand limply and drove off.

Eli had reserved one of the luxury rooms that overlooked the gardens and the pool, and once the bags had been deposited he quickly placed a call to Leslie Robertson. Jo busied herself unpacking and setting up her vital cosmetics in the bathroom.

The call rang through and Leslie's assistant answered. "Commander Robertson's office, this is Dominica speaking. How may I help you?"

"This is Eli Rose speaking. I have a meeting with the Commander for three this afternoon and I just want to confirm that we're still on."

"Just one moment, sir, I'll check," answered his assistant. There was silence for a minute and then she said, "Sir, Commander Robertson says please come over as soon as you are able. He has a few things to discuss with you."

"Very good," answered Eli. "Please tell him I'll be there in an hour. Cheers."

"Jo, I need to go over and see Leslie Robertson right now. Do you mind if I abandon you for a couple of hours?"

Jo came out of the bathroom and smiled. "You're kidding, of course. Remember, I'm your shadow for the next two weeks, so don't even think about ditching me like I'm some silly bimbo just along for the ride." She went back into the bathroom and called out, "You're on the couch tonight."

Eli had already guessed as much, and that was just fine.

"Great. Look, if you're coming with me then we need to leave in half an hour. It will only take a few minutes to get there but I want to stop and get a box of Graycliff Chateau cigars before we go."

"Ready," she announced, emerging from the bathroom in a pair of khaki trousers and a conservative white cotton shirt.

"Wow, very impressive and appropriate for the destination."

She curtsied and smiled. "I'm not completely boorish. I can behave when I want to. After you."

Eli led the way down to the lobby and was able to put the cigars on the room tab. They passed through the narrow entrance and the bellman immediately hailed a taxi.

"We need to go to the RBDF," Eli told the driver.

"De RBDF? You got some trouble, general?" answered the old driver.

"No, just visiting a friend."

"Yea' man, we goin'."

The driver sped off towards Blue Hill Road and once out of central Nassau, drove quickly down to Carmichael Road and out to the west. Eli and Jo sat silently while the old driver pointed out sights of interest, mainly to him, and in a few minutes they had made the turn onto Coral Harbour Road and the entrance to the Royal Bahamian Defense Forces headquarters. Eli could see two of the RBDF's Acklins-class patrol boats at dock, and he wished he could be using one of them to get around instead of the sailboat he'd rented. The big 7.62 mm deck guns might come in real handy if there was trouble.

"Yuz know dat' dis' place were de' Coral Harbour Hotel once upon a time." The old man checked the rearview mirror to gauge the interest of his passengers.

"Really," said Jo, feigning interest. "And what's so special about that?"

"Ah, dey make dat' James Bond movie der'. Ma' cousin were in it."

"Very interesting," Jo replied. She smiled at Eli but he took little notice, preferring to concentrate on the job at hand. He needed to get Leslie's help with logistics and support, especially if anything went wrong. How best to arrange that was his primary concern.

"Here we go," said the old driver as they pulled up to the main building. "Ten dollars." Eli handed him fifteen and the guy said, "Peace be wit' ya', general."

"Follow me," said Eli. He and Jo went into the building and checked with the guard at the reception station. "Eli Rose and friend to see Commander Robertson," he said to the guard.

The guy dialed the office number and then said, "Please go to five, sir. His assistant will meet you there."

They took the elevator up and when the doors opened a pretty young girl greeted them.

"You must be Mr. Rose, and guest. I am Dominica, Commander Robertson's assistant. Please come with me." Dominica accompanied them to the office and Leslie welcomed them in.

"Eli, you old dog. So good to see you." The two men shook hands warmly.

"Leslie, it's been a long time but you haven't aged a bit. And you've made Commander. Congratulations. When did that happen?"

"Last year, thanks to you. And who is this beautiful person with you?"

"Jo McHenry, this is my good friend Leslie Robertson. Leslie, Jo McHenry."

"It's a pleasure to meet you, Leslie," said Jo shaking his hand.

"No, the pleasure is definitely mine," Leslie replied. "Eli, you're traveling in better company these days."

"Watch out for this one, Jo," said Eli with a wink. "He's quite the ladies man."

Leslie laughed and Jo just smiled, so Eli continued quickly.

"So Leslie, you obviously got my message. What do you have for me?"

The Commander called out for Dominica to hold his calls. "Would you like a drink? I'm afraid we have no alcohol here, but I can offer you a cold Club Soda."

"That would be great," said Jo. Dominica entered a few seconds later with a bottle and a cup with some ice.

"Thank you Dominica. Now, Eli, regarding your request. I'm afraid I have some bad news for you. So far, we haven't been able to locate the boat or the two people in question. But we do have some interesting leads that you may want to follow up."

Leslie paused for a moment to sip his own drink. He was only thirty three and already well placed within the RBDF. Eli admired his well pressed uniform and was happy to see that Leslie acknowledged his help in gaining his promotion. Tipping him off had led to the seizure of that drug mother ship, and Leslie received credit for one of the largest drug busts in Bahamian history. Now, as head of the Intelligence Branch, he was in a great position to help with any number of problems that might fall out of Eli's investigative activities in the area.

"My friend, everything I'm about to tell you is purely unofficial. Please don't make any of it public."

"Of course not."

"Very good. So we did some asking about in the Berry's and the Abaco's and didn't get much we could use. But we checked with some local fishermen in Andros Town and one of them remembered seeing a boat like the one you described, a Morgan Out Islander of about forty feet or so, tied up off the beach at the Joulters Cays. He thought it was strange because almost no one goes there."

"That's a great lead," said Eli with relief. "We can start there."

"Hold on. There's more you should know. This is highly confidential, but we've been dealing with some acts of piracy in that area for the past few months, and so far we haven't been able to catch the buggers. Our fast boats patrol the area when they can and we send over the *Andros* and the *Abaco* when we can, but so far we haven't been able to stop them. The word around town is that they are a group from Shower Posse that have gone out on their own. We can't let this get out because it will not be good for tourism and I don't want to have to explain it to anyone in Government. You understand?"

"Absolutely," said Eli. "We won't let it get out." He looked over at Jo, who sat with her arms folded and was obviously unhappy.

Leslie noted her distress and added, "Miss McHenry, please understand. I am not saying your parents were the victims of pirates or drug runners. We don't even know if that was their boat. We see hundreds of similar vessels in the area of the Berry Islands every week. It could have been anyone."

"Thank you Commander," said Jo. "I understand, but it doesn't look good. Please excuse me. I need some air."

The two men stood up as Jo exited the room. Eli was about to follow her but Leslie grabbed his arm and motioned for him to stay.

"Eli, we need to talk about this a bit more. I don't approve of you going out there to look for these people without help. I can't order you to accept it, but you'd be foolish to turn me down."

"Leslie, you said that you didn't have much luck turning up leads. When your uniformed guys show up all the locals go quiet. I won't have any better luck if I have a couple of your guys with me. It will be obvious as soon as we hit Andros Town." He patted his friend on the shoulder.

"No, we're going alone. We can blend in with the rest of the tourists that way and maybe a few discreet questions about our "friends" will get some results.

Now, were you able to do the other thing I asked you to do?"

Leslie shook his head and sighed. "You really are extraordinary, you know. Yes, my men have been on your rental and installed the special "equipment" you requested. That was bloody touchy, by the way."

Eli smiled and got up. "I knew you could do it," he said with a smile. So the plan is a go for tomorrow. We're off to Andros Town and now it looks like we'll spend a second day searching the Joulters. We should be back in Nassau no later than Monday, even if we take a day off to do some fishing. If we're not back by then, send the cavalry."

"Right, my friend." Leslie gave Eli a bear hug and a pat on the back. "We'll be watching for you."

Eli turned to leave but stopped as he opened the door. "Oh yes, I almost forgot. When we were walking into the building I found this lying on the ground out front. It's strange that someone would leave a box of such good cigars for just anyone to pick up." Eli handed the box to Leslie. "I'll turn these in to you. I trust you'll know what to do with them."

Leslie smiled and took the box. "It's a good thing I don't have any political aspirations. God knows what would turn up just lying around."

Chapter 8

The ringing startled Vicente. He reached for his alarm and knocked it off the nightstand trying to turn it off. But the ringing continued - it was the telephone!

"Who is calling at this hour," he cursed aloud to himself. He grabbed the receiver and calmed himself before answering. "*Si*."

"The meeting will be at eight this morning under the I-95 overpass. Go to the parking lot where Northwest North River Drive runs into Southwest 3rd Street. Go alone." The voice on the other end did not wait for a reply and the line went dead.

Vicente cursed again and swung his feet off the bed. He had more than enough time to make the meeting; it was just five in the morning. But he needed a couple of *café cubanos* to get his head straight first. He showered quickly and dressed in a casual tan *guayabera* with matching linen trousers. He selected his brown, hard-toed Kenneth Cole shoes just in case he had to use them for something other than walking, and slipped his short-blade stiletto into its case. The guy that sold it to him designed it to hang from his neck like a gold chain, just over his sternum. No one could see what was there, just under his shirt. As always, it was a last resort, one he'd thankfully only had to use once.

He drove over to the Las Brisas Cafetería, not because he liked the place but because it was one of the few that was open at six-thirty in the morning. The food was passable and the coffee acceptable, so he sat at a small table in the corner and read his copy of *El Nuevo Herald* while he had his *cafecitos* and a couple of meat-filled *pastelitos*.

At seven-thirty he drove to the parking lot under the I-95 overpass and got out of the Corvette. He leaned against the door and waited. He knew he'd been watched since he turned onto 3rd Street, but that was to be expected. Once they felt he was alone the meeting would begin. Vicente looked at his watch. Eight o'clock. He would wait only five more minutes; any longer and he would appear too anxious. Just as he was about to leave he saw a pair of black Chevy Suburbans approaching from North River Drive. *So it begins*, he thought.

The vehicles pulled into the parking lot and quickly boxed him in, one just a few feet in front of the Corvette and the other at a similar distance behind. Seven young, well-dressed *Cubanos* exited the vehicles and formed up on either side of him.

"You know the drill," said one of the guys with long, black hair, and Vicente raised his arms and leaned over onto his car. The guy stepped up quickly and frisked has back and legs, then pulled him around and frisked his arms and waistband. The guy was thorough -

he checked under Vicente's arms, his upper thighs, his ankles. When he was satisfied that the old man was not carrying a weapon he waved to the Suburban in front and another guy got out and approached the group.

"He's clean," said the young guy that had done the search.

"Ok, very good. Thanks, Rudy." The guy turned to face Vicente and said to him in street Spanish, "So I get a call at midnight from a guy that I know and he says some big shot wants to meet me. Says I can't blow him off because he's got connections. That really pissed me off old man. I don't like to be pushed into anything. You better be worth it or I'll be driving that nice little Stingray of yours home tonight."

Vicente sized him up and smiled. So this was Paco Gutiérrez. He was not a physically impressive guy; shorter than Vicente and thin, not muscular at all. *Probably no older than twenty five*, he thought, *probably a Colombiano based on his accent.* He definitely dressed the part of a drug dealer, right down to the ponytail and Ray-Ban sunglasses. *A good looking kid*, thought Vicente. *I hope his mother loves him.*

The old man bowed slightly and answered in formal Spanish. "My name is Vicente Amarón, at your service. Maybe you heard of me, maybe not. But I am the person you need to talk to about your import business."

Paco laughed and slapped his young body guard on the shoulder. "Rudy, you hear this asshole? He wants to talk to me about my "import" business." He walked up to within a few inches of Vicente's face and growled, "What business did you say, asshole? What business do you think I have? And who the hell needs you?"

"You are importing cocaine from Cuba, *Señor* Gutiérrez. You transfer cargos from Colombia to Miami using the port at Cardenas. You have protection from certain officials in the government, this much I know about your business. But I also know from my sources that the Cuban government has started an investigation of your friends and that you have had to look for alternate means of "importing" your products until the situation cools down. That's where I can help you."

The young guy backed away and studied Vicente for a moment. "How do you know all of this, old man?"

"As I told you, I have my sources."

"You have your sources. Well then, maybe you are gonna' tell me who are your sources so I can find out how they know about this." He waved for Rudy and another guy to stand on either side of Vicente. "Now, because you are an old man and I'm a sympathetic guy, I will make you a deal. You tell me everything I want to know and you can leave in one piece. You try and get cute with me and Alvaro here will cut off your ear. That will hurt a lot and I wouldn't advise it. You also might have a problem hearing my questions."

Alvaro was a big guy, and Vicente was not happy about having to deal with him. Alvaro stood to Vicente's left and pulled a large buck knife from his coat pocket and held it to his left ear.

"So what's your choice, old man?" said Paco. "You talk or do we start cutting pieces off you?"

Vicente smiled broadly and turned slowly to face Alvaro, making him reach out with his left arm to keep the knife in place. In one lightning fast motion, Vicente shot his right hand up and grabbed Alvaro's wrist, pulling it away from his ear, while he slammed the palm of his left hand up and under the guy's nose. Stunned, Alvaro dropped the knife and fell backwards against the Corvette. Before Rudy could grab Vicente, the older man kicked out with his left foot, contacting his attackers groin with pinpoint accuracy. Rudy collapsed to his knees with both hands cupped over his genitals while Vicente picked up the knife. As he turned around he heard the distinctive click of a safety being turned off.

Paco stood there with his arm outstretched, holding a Glock 9 millimeter that was pointed at Vicente's forehead.

"Wow, very impressive," he said with a grin. "You may be an old man but your pretty fast. Maybe not like Superman, not faster than a speeding bullet. What you think?"

"What I think," gasped Vicente, trying to catch his breath, "is that my contacts will only work with me, so you are wasting your time and all this is for nothing." He pulled a handkerchief from his pocket to dab up the blood coming from the small cut next to his ear. *I'm getting old*, he thought.

Paco lowered his arm and holstered his pistol, then waved at Vicente.

"Let's you and me take a little walk." He put his hand up when his men began to move with him and said, "Guys, stay here and help those morons. We have some private business to discuss."

The pair walked over to the edge of the Miami River and stared at the boats on the other side. They were an odd couple indeed; Vicente, much taller and much older and Paco, young and trendy but as short and thin as a reed.

"So, *Señor* Amarón, what are you proposing to do for me?"

Vicente knew his lines well and spoke convincingly. "First, because I will provide you with a safe route for your "cargoes," I want ten percent of your gross sales to third party dealers. I also need a cash advance - fifty thousand dollars up front because I have to pay some people to set up the drops. That's all."

The young guy put his hands on his hips and then waved his arms.

"That is fucking outrageous. Ten percent of the gross - nobody gets that."

"Not until now," said Vicente. He grinned and added, "I will even throw in a receiving station in Mexico, just because I like you so much."

At this the young guy burst out laughing and grabbed Vicente's arm.

"You are so full of bullshit. Ok, it's a deal. You can't audit me, but if you do what you say I'll honor the deal."

"Great," Vicente replied, ready to shake his hand.

But Paco's expression turned sour and he grabbed Vicente's arm harder.

"But if you lie to me, or something goes wrong, there won't be enough left of you to put into a Ziploc bag. Understand?"

Vicente pulled his arm free but kept smiling. "I understand, *amigo*."

"One more thing - I'm gonna' have my people check

you out, here and in Cuba. If they come up with anything that that don't jive with your story, you're dead."

"Don't worry, Paco. Everything will be fine. I will contact you tomorrow so we can plan the first drop. How does that sound?" He extended his hand and looked at his young partner.

Paco shook his hand and forced a cynical smile. "Everyone," he called out to his men. "We have a new partner. Come on, be nice and welcome him to the family." The other guys walked over to shake his hand, including Alvaro, still bleeding from the nose and Rudy, who could not yet stand up straight.

"Vicente, take my card. That is my private number. Use it only for this call tomorrow and in case of an emergency. Only for that, understand?"

"Sure, Paco, I got it. Now, if it's Ok with you, I have many things to arrange so I need to go and make some calls. I will contact you tomorrow morning at about eight."

They shook hands again and Vicente watched the men get back into the Suburbans and speed away.

Vicente maintained his calm exterior because he still suspected he was being watched. He drove back to his apartment and sat down on his sofa. His legs were weak and his hands were shaking, so he carefully poured himself a rum on the rocks and sat back down. *I am getting old*, he repeated to himself. *I am really getting old.*

§

"Rise and shine, boss. It's getting on first light and we need to get going." Eli turned on the light in the bedroom and Jo rolled over, covering her head with a pillow.

"Go away," she moaned.

"I told you not to drink more than one of those Goombays."

"What can I say? I was drowning my sorrows in rum. God I feel terrible. My head is pounding like a steel drum."

"Yeah, it's the sugar from the juice. Let's get some coffee into you and you'll be fine. Come on.......... up." He pulled the covers off her and grabbed her feet. "We really have to go."

"Ok, Ok, I'm getting up. Give me five minutes."

Eli closed the door and finished putting his sea bag together. Everything was there - clothes, protective gear, his maps and compass, plus his trusty Beretta. *The boat should be ready to go*, he thought, provisioned for two weeks even though they should only need a few days. He hoped that Leslie had been able to put his extra "equipment" on board as he'd said he did.

Jo emerged from the bedroom carrying a small waterproof bag and her large hat. Eli literally stood and stared at her when she walked into the room.

"What are you gawking at?" she said, clearly irritated.

"Nothing. Let's go."

Eli could not believe how good she looked. He tried not to think about it, tried not to focus on the obvious, but it was unavoidable. She wore a shorter pair of shorts than the previous day, and the even tan on her long and muscular legs contrasted dramatically with the white fabric. Her loose white cotton blouse was tied at the bottom and barely covered the bikini top she wore underneath. With her long platinum blond hair tied up in a bun and her Persol sunglasses she really looked the part of a rich tourist.

They told the girl at the desk that they would be on a sailing trip for a few days and to continue to hold the room, and then they were off to the Nassau Yacht Haven to pick up the boat.

"We're looking for Terry Banford," said Eli to the guy in the office.

"He's out on de' main dock, der."

"Thanks. Let's go," he said to Jo, half pulling her out the door. He wanted to get under way now that the sun was up because it would take about twelve hours to get to Andros Town, even if everything went smoothly.

They walked out onto the dock and could see only one man working on a sailboat, so Eli and Jo approached him. "Are you Terry Banford?" said Eli.

"You found 'em. And ya' must be Mr. Rose and friend." Banford smiled and shook Eli's hand. He was tanned and his skin was like well-worn leather. With his close-cropped white hair and white T-shirt he stood out starkly against the crystalline blue-green water of the harbor.

"Ready to come aboard?" he asked.

"Sure," said Eli. Banford extended his hand to Jo, who grabbed it and jumped onto the deck smoothly. Eli followed, carrying their bags.

"So this is our boat for the next two weeks?"

"This be her," said Banford. "So welcome aboard de *Bree-zee*. We can stow ya' bags in de forward cabin and then you and me, Mr. Rose, we need to be doin' a review of de equipment before ya' leave."

"Ok. Ready when you are."

"We both are," said Jo, grinning.

"That's fine. So let's first start with de above decks. I know ya' sail before, Mr. Rose. Have ya' sail, mam?"

"Yes, many times with my parents. It was several years ago, but I think I can still remember what to do."

"Very good, very good. So ya' controls and winches are de same as de Morgan ya' tole me 'bout. Dis' one a bit older model, a course. De *Bree-zee* be a 1983 but she's a fine boat. Ya' anchor be here on the winch, ya' have some storage der where we keep the life vests and de safety equipment, and back here in de center cockpit be de controls for de motor." Banford walked them around the boat for a few minutes and then took them below to the cabin.

"So generally, we don't want to use de marine head unless we have to. The engine room be here, but if ya' have a serious problem ya' need to use de VHF to call us. We monitor Channel 16 and Channel 9, so call in if ya' need to. Of course ya' know how to open de hatches. We have a wind sock for de forward hatch if ya' want to use it. I recommend it because Andros Town can be still sometimes, no breeze. De controls for de oven be here and de cook top here. I have de cooler stocked up for ya' and de cans of provisions ya' requested."

"Good, thanks."

"And here, this be where we keep de rest a de safety gear. De fire extinguisher, fully charged; de dry bag, which has ya' flare pistol and eight flares, six hand-held flares, a mirror, a whistle, and all dat. Ya' life preservers be above like a showed ya' and I recommend ya' have dem within easy reach at all times. So, der be anything ya' need to ask me?"

"It's all pretty clear," said Eli. "Jo, any questions?"

"None from me."

"Well then, all ya' charts be laid out and ready, I done a radio check to make sure ya' operational. Ya' tole me ya' know how to use de RDF, so if der be nothing more ya' be free to go. Just make sure ya' follow de channel under de bridge and out pass de end of de island. Stay on de outside until ya' round de point at Goulding, then steer a south-southeast course of one fifty seven degrees until ya' get de signal from de Andros Town beacon, then go due west at two seventy degrees and ya' der."

Eli shook his hand again. "Thanks a lot Mr. Banford. We'll see you in a couple of weeks." He picked up the bags and said to Jo, "Why don't you put these in the aft cabin?"

"I'll put mine in the aft cabin. You can use the forward cabin." She disappeared inside and Eli went in and started the little motor. Jo came back out so he added, "We'll motor out until we're in the cruise ship channel. Then we'll raise the sails and see what she can do."

"That sounds pretty good," said Jo. "Father usually started that way, so I can do that pretty well. Do you want me to crank the mainsail or hoist the Genny?"

"You think you have the arm strength to pull the Genny?"

She shot him a dirty look. "I exercise five days per week and I'm a lot stronger than I look."

"Ok, Ok. No offense intended."

"Good. Then none taken."

The *Bree-zee* was rigged as a ketch, with a main and mizzenmast, and a Genoa rigged to the bowsprit. Eli had sailed on a similar boat when he was younger, with a friend from college whose parents kept it at the Dinner Key Marina. He'd learned a fair amount about how to handle them, but was admittedly rusty. *Thank goodness she's done this before,* he thought. It would definitely be a plus that Jo's experience with her parents meant that she really knew a lot about how to handle these boats.

Jo untied the dock lines and Eli backed the *Bree-zee* out of its berth. He cranked the wheel hard over and they were off, slowly chugging out into Nassau Harbour and towards the channel. There was a good breeze up and the sky was mostly clear - only a few fair weather *cumulus* clouds to interrupt the broiling sun. Jo put on her large floppy hat and Persol's and looked absolutely smashing in the bright sun. Eli put on his Maui Jim's for the water, since they cut the glare better than anything he'd tried, but he had to admit that those Persol's looked *great* on her. She sat down across from him and they stared at the cruise ships as the *Bree-zee* motored by.

Chapter 9

Eli felt pretty good. They'd managed to get away early, so barring anything unusual, they would be in Andros Town before dark. And he began to feel better about the job, too. Maybe what he was trying to do was achievable after all. They had a good lead from the RBDF and support from Leslie's men, plus his boss was turning out to be more of a help than he would have guessed when the job first started. In a way, he couldn't help but admire Jo for her emotional strength in dealing with the disappearance of her parents. It would have been too much for others to bear, and she was holding up remarkably well.

As luck would have it, a Royal Caribbean cruise ship was headed out the channel ahead of them so Eli just steered in behind the huge vessel and followed it out between Arawak and Paradise Islands. Once they had cleared the channel Eli passed the wheel to Jo and said, "You know what to do. Let her take some air close to the wind but not dead on."

He climbed up on deck and went over to the main

mast, loosened and pulled the line from the cleat, and pulled the mainsail up until it was extended. Jo expertly steered out so that the sail filled tightly, and Eli secured the boom and the kicker. Jo then went forward to raise the Genoa with the winch.

She pulled hard around the winch, bracing her feet on the forward hatch and leaning back with the line. The big sail billowed out and she trimmed it in perfectly. She walked back and took a seat beside him.

"Wow, you really are good at this," he said, genuinely impressed.

"I told you, I've been doing this with my parents for years. I'm a bit out of practice but I remember most of it." She smiled, broadly a look of self satisfaction on her face. She crawled around behind him and pulled up the mizzen, cleating it off in one swift motion.

"Just like a pro," exclaimed Eli. "Great job. Let's keep a watch for Goulding Cay. I want to be sure we are outside and don't cut the turn too close."

"Aye, aye, Captain," she replied. "I'm going to get a beer. Can I bring you one?"

"Sure, sounds great."

She went below and emerged a few seconds later with two cold Kaliks and was wearing only her light blue string bikini. Eli almost let go of the wheel when he saw her coming out of the cabin. She handed him a bottle and sat down opposite him with her feet on the cushion, looking across him and out at the island.

"What are you staring at?" she said, lowering her sunglasses to look at him.

"Well, you actually."

"Like what you see?"

He took and deep breath and steadied himself, trying to think of something clever to say. "It's a beautiful day, and you fit the picture perfectly." *Shit, that's all I can think of?* he thought.

"Thanks for the compliment," she said. Jo flipped her sunglasses back down and turned her gaze forward. She grabbed the binoculars and scanned ahead for the last island before the Tongue of the Ocean abyss. "At least I'm starting to feel human again after last night."

The east wind kept the sails filled and they were making almost seven knots, better than Eli expected. The ease of their departure caused his thoughts to drift again to Jo. *My God*, he thought. *She must know how good she looks?* Eli tried not to stare but couldn't help himself. Those legs - long, tanned, muscular, ending at a perfect, heart-shaped rear. *No tan line on those cheeks. She's not afraid to show what she's got*, he thought. Smooth, flat stomach and large, cone-shaped breasts barely contained by the bikini top. Staring at her, thinking about her made him react, so he quickly refocused and stared ahead at the horizon.

"Do you see anything yet?" he asked, hoping she would keep staring ahead and not at him.

"I think so. Yes, there to port at about eleven o'clock. Here, let me take the wheel. You have a look." She handed him the binoculars and slid over beside him before he could move.

Eli slipped to his left and stared out from under the Bimini cover. "Yep, there it is. Steer a heading of two forty five degrees. That should put us well clear of the reef. Once we're west of the island we can tack and go southeast along the bank." He looked back at her, sitting there handling the big wheel, wind blowing through her hair and marveled at how beautiful she was.

"There you go, staring at me again," she said, smiling.

"I'm sorry. It's really unprofessional of me, and I promise I won't do it again. It's just that - and please forgive me because I don't mean this in anything but the best way - you look like some high-fashion model from *Vogue* or one of those magazines. You sitting there behind the wheel - it's just a really stunning picture, that's all."

Jo smiled broadly, clearly pleased with the compliment. "You know, I did that for a living for a couple of years, just after high school," she said. "I was young and stupid and I thought I could make my own way in the world without any help from Mother and Father."

"So what happened?"

She sighed and her expression changed noticeably; the darkness of her Persols prevented Eli from seeing her eyes.

"I developed some really destructive habits, and ended up in a really bad relationship. You know, you're young, you think you're hot stuff and you're making good money. It seems like you can do anything. I got some good gigs early on and some important people said some flattering things, made some good stuff happen for me. But it was an illusion, it was never real. I just thought it was. One day I woke up and realized I'd been pretty stupid about my life, and that was it." Jo kept steering and looked ahead silently.

"Wow, sorry I mentioned it," said Eli, genuinely

concerned. "I didn't mean to dredge up any bad memories."

"Not a problem," she replied. "It's all in the past and I've moved on." She paused for a second and added, "But we are getting along much better now, and I'm happy about that. You seem to have accepted that we're in this together and I appreciate your spirit of cooperation."

"Sure," Eli said. "We aim to please."

Cooperation was certainly the best route to take, but he was still uncomfortable having her come along, especially if things didn't go exactly to plan. The last thing he needed was a liability to keep him from going about his business in the way he knew he must. If everything went smoothly, this would end up as nothing more than a nice cruise, and they'd part company all smiles. She'd get her answers, the check would clear, and Eli would get his million.

"Ok, you see the island?" he suddenly said, pointing to the indistinct little island to his left.

"I got it."

"According to the charts we'll need to wait until it's behind us to turn." He pointed at the folded map, moving close so she could see.

"Ok, you say when." Jo gripped the wheel firmly with both hands and stared ahead intently, like she was driving a Formula 1 racer.

"Hey, relax," said Eli, grabbing her left hand. "No need to use a "death grip" for this."

The touch of their hands was brief but they both took notice. Eli withdrew his hand quickly but Jo looked at her hand as though it had been burned.

"A little further - Ok, cut the wheel over."

The boat turned briskly and the sails flipped until they filled again. The *Bree-zee* leaned hard over to the right, catching the stiff breeze full on. They began to bounce in the swells from the deep water, even though they were close to the shallows, but Jo soon cut the waves expertly and evened out the ride. Eli sat back and watched the compass.

"Ok now, head south-southeast at about one fifty four degrees. I'll keep a watch for this section of coral heads here. That's the last thing we'll need to worry about before we turn west." He showed her the map again and pointed out a shallow area about eight and a half miles away.

"Yes, I see it. You just tell me what to do and I'll drive," she said with a grin.

Eli wondered if that was intended as a double *entendre* or if it was just the way she talked. He decided not to make a comment and continued to stare through the binoculars at the horizon.

"We can stop for lunch when we get to the reef, if you like. We've made good time so far, and if we don't take too long we should make Andros Town by six thirty."

"That would be good," she said. "I'm sure I'll want something by then."

Eli was quiet for most of the next hour while Jo concentrated on keeping the *Bree-zee* as close to the recommended course as possible. The sun shone intensely and the water was clear green to their left, deep azure blue to their right. She had the boat right where he wanted it, and he was satisfied that they would be on schedule.

"We're getting close, now," Eli said, suddenly breaking the silence. "Put her dead in the wind and I'll drop the sails. We'll cruise in on the motor so we have some control around the coral heads."

Jo turned west and the sails suddenly fluttered, gasping for air. Eli rolled in the Genoa, quickly secured it and then dropped the mainsail. He stayed up on the deck and pointed for Joe to head into the shallows, almost due east at their location.

"That's it," he yelled. "Cut the engine." Jo complied and Eli dropped the anchor into a large patch of sea grass. They dragged anchor for a few seconds before the large flukes dug in. He turned to congratulate her but she just sat there with her hands gripped tightly to the wheel.

"Hey, you did great. You can relax now," he said, jumping back down into the cockpit.

She smiled a bit and looked more relieved than excited.

"Yeah, thanks. I haven't done that in awhile." Jo released her grip and rubbed her hands. "How about a bottle of water?"

"I'll get it," said Eli. "Take it easy for a few minutes, then I'll fix us some lunch. We have a little fresh fruit in the cooler, some bread and peanut butter and jam. I'm afraid the rest is out of a can."

"I'm good for now, but the water sounds great."

Eli grabbed a couple of bottles and took a seat across from his boss. She opened the bottle and took a long drink of the cold liquid, sat back and exhaled loudly.

"Oh, that's much better," she said with a smile. "By the way, thanks for being so nice back there and not yelling at me."

"No reason to do that," he said. "You did a fine job, handled her like a real pro."

"Well, thanks just the same. Father would have been screaming orders at the top of his lungs if he'd been here. I would have just melted if it had been him." She seemed sad and sounded more like a wounded little girl than an heiress.

"So your father was pretty tough on you?" queried Eli.

"I guess this is "true confessions" day," she replied. "Maybe it's the setting - sailing in the islands again. It brings back some good and not so good memories."

"Sorry about that," he answered. "I seem to be doing that a lot today. I don't mean to pry, so just forget I said anything."

"No, really. It's Ok. It's just that, Father always saw me as his next in line, even if I didn't always see myself that way. He felt like if he pushed me, helped me to think like a man, like *him*, that it would somehow make me stronger and more capable. We had some fights - really ugly fights. I was that rebellious teenage know-it-all, and he was the classic domineering parent."

"What about your mother? Is she the same or does she ever take your side?"

Jo sighed and sat back, taking another drink. she put her legs up on the cushions and stretched.

"Mother is..........compliant, let's say. She doesn't

stand up to Father very often because Father gives her everything she wants, at least in terms of creature comforts. That always put me on an island with Father when we argued, and when things got hot between me and dear old Dad, she would usually find a reason to be out of the room or out of the house. She's a sweet person, but I think her character is why Father wanted me to be different. He knew I could never run McHenry-Taylor if I turned out like Mother."

"Well don't worry, I'm not your father and I promise I won't act like him, even if I'm old enough to be your father."

The girl lowered her sunglasses and stared at Eli with her cold blue eyes. "That's funny. So for grins, how old do you think I am?" she said.

Eli hated these types of questions from women. These types of queries are all trick questions. Does this make me look fat? Do you think she's pretty? How old do you think I am? He knew he couldn't win. He knew no man could win when he had to answer one of "those" questions.

"Ok, I'll bite. I'd say you're twenty three, maybe." She laughed and he thought, *Well, at least she's not screaming at me.*

"Try twenty six."

"No way," he said. "You look way younger than that."

Jo smiled. She looked happy, a definite change from earlier in the conversation.

"I'll take that as a compliment. Wow, you're just full of compliments today. You must want something from me."

Lady, if you only knew, he thought. "Nope, just trying to be honest. You really look like a kid. Now me on the other hand......"

"You," she replied. "You look maybe, forty or a bit younger. But based on what I know about your history, I'm thinking forty two or forty three."

"Not a bad guess. I'm forty four, but sometimes it feels more like seventy four."

"Forty-four! Hey, you look pretty good yourself."

"Still, I'm old enough to be your father," he said.

She slid over closer to him and said, "Chronologically speaking, that's true. But you do look *really* good for forty four." She slid up next to him and put the water bottle to her lips, caressing the opening with her tongue.

"You've been about as nice to me as any man has for a long time," she purred. "I don't really even know you, but I find you fascinating." She looked into his eyes and he was momentarily hypnotized by her stare.

"You know, I'm used to getting whatever I want, whenever I want it." She leaned forward slightly and reached around her back to untie her bikini top. The strings fell to her sides and the top slipped away, exposing her beautiful tanned breasts.

Eli's heart was pounding and he tried to look away and say something to defuse the situation.

"Jo, I really don't think this is a good.........."

She moved in quickly and kissed him, shooting her tongue into his mouth and grasping his head in her hands. She stayed on the kiss for a few seconds and then pulled away, only inches from his face.

"Jo, we need to be profess............"

She kissed his neck and moved back to his mouth, sliding up to him so she could sit on his lap. She straddled him and felt his reaction through the tiny bikini bottoms she still wore.

"So, you do like me? I was beginning to think that maybe you didn't like girls." Jo buried her tongue in his mouth again and started grinding herself into his groin.

"Jo, you're not giving me any options here," said Eli, struggling not to let himself go.

She pulled back for a second and threw off the bikini top. "Don't you like what you see?" she said. "Tell me you don't like me," she teased.

That was it for Eli, and he succumbed to her ample charms. She sat on his lap and they moved together, slowly at first, then faster. They made love under the Bimini top, careful to stay on the cushions but oblivious to the rest of their surroundings. She groaned loudly and pushed her hips at him, and it took all his effort to keep from losing control. When they were both satisfied, they collapsed on the cushions and lay there quietly for a couple of minutes, soaked in sweat. Jo smiled and touched his face softly and he stroked her neck with his fingers.

Oh, shit, he thought. *I've done it again.* Eli thought he was cured of this behavior, of letting his desires get the better of his judgment. It was a familiar failing for him, and even though he recognized it was in his nature, he also knew that there would be a price to pay for his indiscretion sometime down the road.

Chapter 10

"This is Vicente Amarón. I want to speak with Paco." Vicente's hands were sweating. He tried to steady himself on his sofa but his nervous energy would not permit him to be comfortable.

"Wait," said the heavily accented voice on the phone.

It had taken all night, but Vicente managed to get everything into place. His contacts in Pinar del Río were the most difficult to reach, but he was eventually able to do it through a friend who had a radio. Now all he had to do was convince the young punk that he was the big deal he'd made himself out to be. *That should be easy*, he thought sarcastically to himself.

"Vicente, *amigo*, what's happening?" Paco's whiny, high-pitched voice was unmistakable. "Good that you're punctual. I said eight o'clock and it's eight right now. I like that. So tell me, what's going on?"

"We need to meet, Paco. I no trust the telephone. Then I tell you what you need to know."

There was a moment of silence and then Paco

replied, "Ok, you stand out in front of your building and some of my boys will come over and pick you up in one hour. You Ok with that?"

"Sure, Paco. You are the boss. I am ready in one hour." Vicente heard the receiver click, ending the call.

He gathered his maps and notepad into a manila folder, poured a large rum and put his most comfortable loafers on. He needed the drink, even if it was only eight in the morning. He sat back and tried to let the rum wash over him, wash away his insecurity and fear. He hadn't worked since Nicaragua more than five years earlier, and in the years since he'd spent more time holding a glass than a gun. *Hell, I probably wouldn't even remember how to shoot a gun*, he thought. Just as well. He needed to appear to be less like the foot soldier he really was and more like the senior commander he purported to be, a "leader" of men. Sure, he needed to impress Paco with his local knowledge and contacts, but also with his management skills. He had to look the part *and* act the part.

His hand was shaking. *One more drink.* And that was exactly where he'd ended up after Eli stayed in Costa Rica, at the bottom of a rum bottle, trying to piece together what went wrong. He'd felt abandoned by his friends, even though he'd been the one to break off contact. Was it shame? Embarrassment? His own lack of interest? Vicente didn't know. He only knew that this job with Eli was his last chance at respectability, to regain his reputation and his honor. He had to carry this off. That second drink would have to wait.

Vicente walked down to the covered entrance of his apartment building and stood there with his arms crossed, holding the folder. Within minutes a black Mercedes 560 SEL pulled up and a large guy got out of the back.

"Get in," he said forcefully, and Vicente complied. The guy got into the back seat next to him and they roared off down 8th Street.

"Where we go?" asked Vicente.

The guy next to him sat silently and stared straight ahead.

"Is very far?"

Silence.

"How much time it take?"

"Shut up!" said his companion. "You don talk unless The Boss ask you question."

Vicente recognized the accent. *A Haitian*, he thought. *So Paco will hire anyone if he likes them enough. Good to know.* He was a big guy, but smartly attired in his black suit. His fingernails were trimmed and clean, and he was clean-shaven as well. *Paco likes his people to look good. He doesn't like it when things look out of place. That's also very good to know.*

The car raced down Brickell Avenue and turned onto the Venetian Causeway. They passed over the bridges until they were able to turn onto Di Lido Island and then West Di Lido Drive. The big Mercedes pulled up to a large wrought iron gate and the driver pushed the buzzer to gain entry to the compound.

"*Si?*" was the answer.

"We have the fish," said the driver.

"Ok, pass."

The gates swung open into the compound and they rolled in, circling the drive and stopping in front of the main entrance. Everyone got out and Vicente followed the group to the door. Another buzz and another confirmation of who was requesting access and the doors opened. Vicente was impressed by the amount of control over who was permitted access to the area. It would not be an easy place to visit if you were not expected.

They entered the large living room and Vicente's companion said, "Wait here." He walked out to the back patio through a large sliding glass door while the other three men kept Vicente in view. The large Haitian reappeared and said, "You come," waving his hand for emphasis. The two walked out onto the patio and found Paco shirtless, sitting with five bikini-clad *Latinas*. Their long hair blew gently in the morning breeze, filling the air with the smell of jasmine and vanilla.

"And the man himself arrives. Welcome Vicente. Can I offer you something? An orange juice or a croissant, or maybe something young and sweet?" Paco waved his arm over the girls and they smiled obediently.

"An orange juice would be fine," Vicente replied. "You have a beautiful home here. Thank you for seeing me this morning."

"No, *amigo*, it is I who should thank you. You have come here to solve all my problems, isn't that right? Girls, this man, he makes miracles happen." Paco put his orange juice down and waved at the scene around him.

"Yes, this place is pretty nice. It's a fringe benefit of my line of work. Putting my cash flow to a good use you could say." He turned to the girls and said, "Ok, you all go play for awhile so us men can talk business. Go on, go on. Paco will be with you very soon." The girls got up with their drinks and walked off towards the pool. Paco patted the rear of the girl nearest to him and said, "I have something special for you later." She smiled and gave him a kiss on the cheek.

Paco poured the orange juice for Vicente and sat back in his well padded chair. "So old man, I got back some answers on your background check. Very interesting results." He sat silently for a second and sipped his orange juice, staring at Vicente like he was contemplating what to do about him.

Vicente started to sweat but smiled thinly and tried to stay calm. *He knows something*, he thought. *He knows about the office. He knows about the McHenry case. He knows something*!

"You are a pretty bad dude. At least that's what people here and in Cuba are saying about you. You did some pretty hairy shit back in the day." Paco paused and put his glass down. "I like that. I like that you're not afraid to get dirty when you need to. I think you'll be a good guy to have around." He reached out and the shook hands, this time in a much more civil way.

"Welcome to the team, Vicente. Now tell me, what have you got for me this morning?"

Vicente buried his emotions and kept the same thin smile. Inwardly he was so relieved he almost passed out. He pulled the maps from his folder and said, "May I put the maps on the table?"

"Alvaro, Tony - clear this shit off the table so we can talk." Two of the bodyguards rushed over and began removing the trays of food and the plates. "Ok, got enough space now?"

Vicente spread the maps out in order of presentation, first laying out his map of Yucatán and then his map of Pinar del Río.

"Paco, this is what I have arranged, if you decide to do it. You must first get the shipments to Cuba. If you can do this, the cargoes can be transferred here, on the western point." He pointed to a place on the map that was completely overgrown, save for a small bay.

"The area is a tidal swamp full of mangroves and mosquitoes. The only people in the area live here, to the south in Las Tumbas. This is a curious place that very few people know about. You see, in the old days, the Soviets had a small submarine base here."

Paco burst out laughing and his bodyguards chimed in, grinning at one another and chuckling.

Vicente paused and looked at him, puzzled by his reaction. "There is something funny I do not understand?"

"Old man, you are proving to be a very smart guy. I knew I liked you when I met you. What's so funny you ask? I'll tell you - how do you think we get the drugs up to Cuba in the first place?" He waited for Vicente to ask but when he didn't, Paco continued.

"About six months ago we bought a decommissioned Russian sub. It's an OSKAR-I Class nuclear job. We bought the officers and crew along with the boat. The Russians had already stripped out all of the missile and torpedo gear, but that was better for us. We have amazing space now. We can ship about twenty tons of cocaine at a time and this baby can do fifty days submerged without having to surface for air. Of course, we trimmed the crew to just what we need to run the thing, but so far it has worked perfectly. And if anyone asks, the visits are just a routine stopover."

Vicente was dumbstruck. He suspected such a thing was possible but never dreamed it could really be done.

"This is true? You really have this thing? My God, now I understand."

"Unfortunately, our Cuban Admiral seems to have got himself in a bind with Fidel, so we need to look for another place to land the sub so we can transfer the cargoes to other destinations."

"Yes, this is perfect," said Vicente. "Look, right here there is a long dock that was used by the Soviets to dock the same type of submarines. It is about one hundred fifty meters long, just what you need, I think. I have already confirmed that we can use it after some minor repairs. There is a warehouse just here under the trees and you can store everything there while you wait for your other transportation to arrive."

"Vicente, this is exactly what we needed." Paco leaned over and studied the map, smiling. "I am impressed, old man. You came highly recommended and so far I am impressed. What else do you have?"

Vicente moved the Cuba map over and pulled out the map of Yucatán.

"Again, you must provide the transportation, but here is the destination. This little place is called Chiquilá, and they have a small commercial dock and some warehouses. They are connected to the main highway network so you can bring in trucks and take your drugs wherever you want in just a couple of days."

Paco laughed and slammed his hand down on the map and said, "Old man, you really do have this shit figured out. We've been talking to the Gulf Cartel for a couple of months about doing something just like this, but we couldn't bring the sub into Mexican waters. There's just no place to dock it. This will work out great. We'll use one of our Panamanian cargo carriers to pick up the load in Cuba and transport the stuff there. I can make a deal with the Gulf boys to take it off our hands at the docks and then we don't have to worry about it. They've got the expertise to do this in Mexico, so why not let them? This is great. I can set up my end in a few days. When can you be ready to start?"

"Well, I must coordinate the repair of the facilities in Pinar, but maybe one week?"

Paco sat back and rubbed his smooth chin. "One week. If you can promise me one week then we can do it. I will need to get on a plane for Reynosa tomorrow to make this happen."

"You have the authority to do something like this?" Vicente was curious just how far Paco could go without approval from Medellín.

The little guy got up and leaned on the table, moving close to Vicente's face. "Look, old man, just because maybe I like you and you checked out Ok don't give you any right to question me, understand?"

"*Si*, my friend, I understand. I am only concerned about the timing. If you must go to Medellín then I am thinking this will take more than one week." Vicente was sweating now and his legs were weak. He struggled to maintain control but did not show it outwardly.

Paco stood up and folded his arms, staring coldly at Vicente.

"Alvaro, tell Rudy to get me the telephone. I need to call Pablo, right now."

He just stood there, silently staring at Vicente while skinny Rudy ran back to the house and returned with the mobile telephone. Alvaro's nose was bandaged and his eyes were black and blue from the blow he'd suffered from Vicente, and he glared at him with obvious resentment.

"Call Medellín. Tell them I want to talk with Pablo."

Rudy punched in the number and frowned at Vicente while he watched. He was afraid he'd pushed Paco just a bit too hard and now the guy felt he had to prove that *he* had the appropriate stroke for the job.

"*Si, si.* Paco Gutiérrez calls from Miami. He wants to speak to *Don* Pablo. Ok, Ok." Rudy turned to Paco and said, "One second. They transfer the call." He listened on the other end and then said excitedly, "*Si, si,* boss. Here he is." He shoved the phone at Paco, who gave Rudy a dirty look.

"*Si Don* Pablo. Very good to hear your voice. Oh, so you are down at the ranch. Good, good. *Don* Pablo, the reason for my call is that we have a business opportunity opening up with the Gulf Cartel boys. We can move maybe twenty tons per month through them. No, we haven't discussed the price yet. Oh, thank you very much, *Don* Pablo. You can rely on me to get you the best deal. Oh, thank you *Señor,* thank you. Yes, you also." Paco thrust the phone at Alvaro, who trotted back off to the house with it.

"So, old man, you need more proof I can do what I say I can?"

He was pretty mad, so Vicente paused for a second to be sure to say just the right thing.

"*Señor* Gutiérrez, it has always been clear to me that you are the most important man to talk to in Miami. I never question this. My desire is to help you be successful and for the operation to move without any problems. In order to do this we must have very precise timing, and that is the reason I ask the question. In this way, we can both be very successful."

Paco smiled and then patted Vicente on the shoulder.

"Ok, Vicente. So here's your chance to be a hero. Get the dock and warehouse facilities ready in one week. Contact your people in Chiquilá and make sure we have the space available when the ship gets in. It will take another day to load up and make it over there, so they should be ready to receive the cargo in nine days. I don't want any screw-up's and no excuses, got it?"

"*Si Señor.*"

"Good, good." Paco's attention turned to the girls sitting by the pool. "I think maybe you earned a little extra bonus this morning. Why don't you come over and pick one out for yourself? You can choose any of them that you like. What do you say?" He smiled and put his arm around Vicente's shoulder.

The older man smiled thinly and said, "Maybe next time, Paco. I must get in touch with everyone and get things moving. We do not have much time and there are many things to do."

Paco nodded and grinned. "Ok, maybe next time. I bet an old guy like you could really tear up one of those sweet *chicas*." Alvaro came back from the house and stood at Paco's side with his hands behind his back.

"Listen, I gotta' get this deal done with the *Mexicanos* so I'll be away until Tuesday or Wednesday," said Paco. "You call Rudy here if there is any problem, understand? And remember - I don't expect you to call him." Paco shook Vicente's hand and held on for an extra few seconds.

"You call me on Wednesday and let me know where we are with this. Everything works out, you'll be a very rich man." He waved to Alvaro, who handed him a bulging, legal-sized envelope.

"Here's the "loan" you wanted. Just make sure I get what I'm paying for."

Vicente smiled again and nodded. He just wanted to get the hell out of there before he said something wrong, so he collected his maps and the envelope and waved goodbye to the girls. Paco's men escorted him back to the Mercedes and they were on their way back to Little Havana in an instant.

They left him at the entrance to his building, in the same place where they'd picked him up two hours before. It was only ten o'clock but Vicente was exhausted. There was no time to relax, at least while so much needed to be done. If it was managed just right, he could get the answers he needed, alert the Coast Guard about the shipment to Mexico, and get Paco put away all at the same time. Or, if things didn't work out, he'd be fish food like Julio said. *The little punk is right.*

No screw-up's on this one, he thought.

Chapter 11

"Come in, the water feels great," called Jo. She'd jumped in without her bikini after Eli had tied off a safety line and a float on the rear rail.

"I will. Don't let go of the line. The current is pretty fast here." He jumped over the side and stripped off his bathing suit, throwing it back onto the deck.

Jo moved over to him, put her arms around his neck and wrapped her long legs around his waist. She kissed him again and hugged him tightly.

"That was amazing," she whispered, as if someone was listening. "I've never felt anything like that before, with anyone else. I knew you were special when you came over to the house the other day." She hugged him again and then grabbed the line.

"I'll go make us some lunch. Don't be too long."

Jo pulled herself back to the boat along the line and climbed up the ladder. Eli's gaze was transfixed on her rear, and he marveled at her flawless skin tone and smooth, even tan. He felt a new surge of interest course through him, but quieted his thoughts to focus on the rest of the crossing. They still needed another two hours sailing south to get to their crossing point, and then it was a straight sail west to get to Andros Town. He would look for a signal from the radio direction finder when they had sailed about an hour and a half, since the crossing would probably take about three hours. That should put them in at about six in the afternoon, and they could then anchor out in Fresh Creek and use the dingy to go to town. He pulled himself to the boat and pulled in the line and float.

"Lunch is served," said Jo. She had put her bikini back on before she came back up on deck, and carried a tray with a couple of sandwiches, some crackers, and bottled water. "What a great view," she said with raised eyebrows as she gazed at Eli.

He hadn't put his suit back on yet so he replied, "Well, take a good look because you won't be getting a peak again until later tonight."

She frowned, feigning disappointment. "If you insist. But I'll need another look later, because that just wasn't enough."

Eli smiled and pulled on his bathing suit. They ate quickly and drained the water before getting ready to go.

"Let's take a second to go over the float plan," he said, laying out the map. "We're here, and we need to get down to about this spot before we turn west. I figure it will take us about another two hours on the same heading, then we'll turn and I'll guide you in from there."

"Sounds like a good plan to me," she said. "Tell me

when you're ready and we'll get going."

"Ok, you drive. Crank up the engine and let's take some slack up on the anchor line. I'll wave when I've broken it free, and you can turn back southeast until I have it stowed. Then we'll raise the sails."

Jo gave a mock salute and Eli smiled and went up to the bow. When the anchor line went slack he pulled up hard and broke the flukes free of the grassy bottom. He cranked up the windlass and secured the anchor rode and waved at Jo to turn southeast. She used the wind expertly to fall off to starboard and Eli raised the mainsail and the mizzen. He took over from Jo while she raised the Genoa and then handed her back the wheel for the journey south.

Jo kept the *Bree-zee* on the wind and the boat laid over to starboard again. It made for a bumpy ride, but they gained speed and soon were back at seven knots. Eli took the opportunity to go below decks and see if Leslie's men had delivered the special "equipment" he'd requested before they arrived in Nassau. He searched the kitchen storage first but then realized that would be too obvious a place to hide something. He went forward and looked at the storage under the bunk and found it, wrapped in a burlap sack.

Just what the doctor ordered, he said to himself. A new British L85A1 assault rifle, modified for marine use and complete with two extra fifty round magazines. *That will do just fine,* he thought. With his Beretta 92F and the L85 he had enough fire power to hold off any pirates they might run into. He spent quite a bit of time checking out both weapons, making sure they were clean and fit to fire in case he needed them. He also went over the maps again, memorizing the approaches to Andros Town and the area north to Joulters Cay. Before he left the cabin, Eli chambered the first round in the L85 and clicked on the safety. *Ready! Hope I don't need it.* He put the weapons into the side storage locker across from the galley and went back to the cockpit.

The chronometer on Eli's Seiko diving watch showed that a little more than two hours had passed, so he asked Jo to take a break from steering and get some rest. She stretched out on the cushion beside him and laid her head in his lap. She looked up at him and smiled, and he thought that she looked happy for a change. Maybe it was his imagination or just a hangover from their love making, but he felt............happy, too.

"Ok, I'm coming about," he said, turning the wheel to his right. The boat swung over and the sails fluttered and flapped until he caught the wind.

The *Bree-zee* headed off towards the afternoon sun and they had following seas because of the strong east wind, so the boat rolled gently in the swells as they made wake west. Eli trimmed up the sails and they were soon out in deep water, cruising over the deep blue abyss of the Tongue of the Ocean. Jo dozed while Eli kept watch with the binoculars, looking for boat traffic or any signs of land. A small thunderstorm was rolling in from behind them and Eli hoped it would be brief. The ensuing downdraft chilled the air, waking Jo.

"What's that?" she asked with a shiver. She stuck

her head up over the edge of the cockpit and saw the storm. "I better close the hatches," she said, jumping up and heading below. She soon returned wearing a windbreaker and huddled up next to Eli.

"You didn't bring any rain gear?" she asked.

"Nope. It doesn't bother me much," he lied.

"Let me come close - I'll cover you."

"Don't worry about it."

The rain began to fall, slowly at first and then in a great torrent with large, cold drops. Jo nearly crawled on top of Eli to try and cover both of them with her rain jacket and only succeeded in making sure they were both soaked when the sudden downpour had ceased. She went back to the cabin and returned carrying a large beach towel.

"I found this in the bathroom. Nice of them to think of it," she said, drying herself off. "Your turn."

She handed the towel to Eli, who dried his arms and torso and handed it back. "Thanks. Can you handle her for a while? I need to crank up the RDF and see if we can get a signal into Andros Town." He slid out to his left and she slipped in behind the wheel. Jo grabbed the binoculars and had a quick scan of the horizon while Eli went below.

He turned on the old Bendix 550A Radio Direction Finder unit and increased the volume control. He rotated the tuning dial until he could hear a loud beep from the signal in Andros Town.

"Steer a heading of two seventy four degrees," he called up to Jo.

"Ok. Two seventy four degrees."

Eli turned the unit off and came back to the cockpit. Jo continued to steer a smooth course, angling over the swells at times to flatten out the ride but staying close to the heading they needed. Eli scanned the horizon with the binoculars and saw nothing. There was not another boat anywhere around for miles. He could see how easy it would be for the McHenrys to be lost at sea in this area, and he realized that they might never find them or any trace of where they'd been. Eli looked over at Jo, who seemed at peace behind the wheel of the big boat. *I hope she can handle not knowing what happened*, he thought.

He continued to scan the horizon for another few minutes before going below to get another signal from the RDF. He heard the loud beeping of the Andros Town station and came back up to sit with Jo.

"Steer two seventy now. We should be seeing some land on the horizon any time."

Eli grabbed the binoculars, straining to see anything ahead and soon he could see the large clouds that build up every summer afternoon over the warm, shallow waters of the Great Bahama Bank.

"I can see it," he said with some relief. "I have trees on the horizon. Let me get one more bearing and then we'll go by line of sight. Here, hang onto the map. I'll be right back."

His final check of the RDF showed they were right on course. "Maybe another forty five minutes," he said, looking at his watch. They were at the three-hour mark in the crossing, so the wind and current had pushed them farther south then he'd planned. But they would still make Fresh Creek just a few minutes past six, so no damage done.

As they neared the island, Eli scanned the shore for two landmarks that would help him find his destination: the large complex of buildings that marked the AUTEC facility, and the settlement on the north side of Andros Town.

"Ok, we're going to need to turn a bit north," he said. Let's get closer in first and I'll tell you when."

Jo gripped the wheel tightly and her gaze was fixed straight ahead.

"Ok, there's AUTEC. I see their channel - can you see it?"

"Not really," she replied. "The glare off the water is getting bad, so maybe you should take over."

He could tell she was getting nervous but it was a good chance for Eli to show his confidence in her, so he said, "No, you're taking her in. I'll navigate, you drive."

"If you're sure," she said, looking over at him.

He nodded and smiled. They sailed north and passed the AUTEC channel and Eli decided to lower the sails.

"Turn her dead on. I'm going to lower the main and the Genny."

Jo steered northeast to allow the sails to drop air, and Eli lowered the main. He rushed forward and cranked in the Genoa, then quickly came back and turned on the engine before lowering the mizzen.

"Ok, we're on the motor the rest of the way in." He stayed up near the mainmast and called out directions until they were close to the first small island that marked the north edge of the channel.

"Turn hard left and then point the bow towards the

middle of the channel." They motored slowly in until she could see the opening to Fresh Creek.

"I see it now," she said. They continued into the mouth of the river, past the lighthouse and the ferry docks.

"We'll anchor out over there," said Eli, pointing to a spot just away from the main channel. "Come in slowly and then stop and reverse when I tell you."

Jo complied and Eli let the anchor down. They quickly caught and Jo shut down the engine.

"Congratulations, boss," said Eli shaking her hand. "We made it, and you did great."

She shook his hand and then hugged him, pressing tightly against him. "Thank you so much for this," she said tearing up. "No one has ever..........I mean I've never had such a good time with a man before." She hugged him again and kissed him long and deeply.

"It means everything to me that you agreed to take me with you."

"Jo, it's not like you gave me a choice. The way I remember it, you pretty much said either you go or you get someone else to do this job. That was a definite motivation for me to bring you along."

She looked indignant and said, "So that's the only reason you brought me? Because I made you bring me?"

Eli tried to find a good way out so he simply said, "You know that was the deal. But now that we're here I can say that it was great having you with me. If I'd known then what I know now I would have asked you rather than the other way around. That's especially true if I had known that the "fringe benefits" were so fantastic."

She smiled and nodded. "Ok, that's a good answer. Just keep in mind, those "fringe benefits" aren't something my employees ever get to experience. You are the first."

"Trust me, I loved every minute of it. I would never take you for granted."

"Good," she said, hugging him again. "And if you're really nice maybe I'll award you a new set of "benefits" tonight." She slipped her hand into his bathing suit and gasped.

"Oh my God, you have to be kidding me."

"Sorry, boss, but that's what you do to me." He was a little embarrassed but very happy to feel her soft touch.

"It's quite a compliment. I like it. But I think we better secure everything for the night and go ask the questions we need to ask before it gets dark."

"You bet. Can you tie down the mizzen while I take care of the main?"

"Yes, Captain."

They worked for a few minutes to tie down the canvas and then Eli mounted the wind sock to the hatch that covered the rear compartment. They'd need it later when the wind died down and the mosquitoes came out. He set up the mosquito netting and moved his bag into the rear cabin.

"I'm going to put on something respectable," said Jo and she went below.

Eli got the Beretta and an extra clip and set them on the counter in the galley. When Jo had finished, he threw on a shirt and a pair of shorts, shoved the pistol into his belt and grabbed a pair of sandals.

"Let's put the raft in the water and then we can head out. You take that side and I'll take this one."

They lifted the small raft over the side and Eli tied the safety line and float to it.

"Let me get in and see if this motor works first," he added. He climbed down the ladder and got into the raft. Eli choked the little Evinrude motor and pulled hard on the rope. It sputtered to a start on the first try, so he called out, " Come on in and let's go." Jo climbed down the ladder and into the raft. She untied the line and Eli steered the little craft over to the ferry dock. Jo tied them off to a piling and Eli helped her up to the dock. He climbed up and they walked over to the ferry office to see what they could learn.

"Good afternoon, sir, mam," said the cheerful agent at the desk. "Welcome to Andros Town. How can I help you?"

"Hi there. Well, the Missus and I are cruising around the islands for a couple of weeks and we thought we'd come by and see what Andros is all about." Eli shook the guy's hand while Jo looked on, a bit taken aback by the fabrication.

"What's to do around here, I mean besides watery things?"

The clerk smiled and said, "Well, we have some interestin' attractions in de' area. Here's a map dat shows where most of dem are." He unfolded a map and pointed several locations out to Eli.

"Looks interesting," said Eli. "We were hoping to meet up with some friends here. Maybe they stopped in to visit you - the McHenrys? They have a boat like ours called the *Madeleine*. Did you also show them some good places to visit?"

The clerk looked up at Eli for a moment and thought. "Hmm, I don't know those names. You know, we have many people stoppin' here. Sometimes I don't remember who dey are. But der was an older couple here for a night, back about a month ago. They don't stay so I don't get to talk to 'em much. I tink dey went north when dey left."

"Oh, too bad for us I guess. Say, do you know where we can get a taxi around here?"

"Just out de' front be a taxi. Enjoy de' day." The guy smiled and waved as they walked out the front of the building.

Just as the agent had said, a highly used taxi sat by the entrance with its engine off. The driver was napping soundly, snoring away when Eli and Jo walked up. Eli tapped on the roof.

"Hey, friend, you busy?"

"No, general. I be waitin' for ya." The old guy straightened up on his beaded seat as the couple got into the back. "Where ya' wanna' be goin?"

"Take us to the AUTEC front gate." Eli looked at Jo, who looked back and shrugged.

"Yeah, man, we goin."

The old guy started up his equally old Chevy Impala. It sounded like a tank due to a blown muffler, so they rumbled off loudly south and in a minute were at the perimeter fence for the AUTEC facility.

"This is fine," said Eli. "Here's a five. Thanks for the lift."

"Oh, ya' very welcome, general."

They got out and walked over to the one of the SP's guarding the gate. Jo again looked at Eli quizzically but said nothing.

"Seaman, can you do me a favor and call Lieutenant Commander Barnes and tell him Eli Rose is here to see him."

"Is he expecting you, sir?" said the young SP.

"It's a surprise," said Eli, looking at Jo.

"Please wait here while I call." He walked off to the guard shack while the other SP looked on with keen interest.

"Eli, what the hell are we doing here? What is this place?" Jo was pretty agitated but she stayed composed, not knowing what was going on.

"Welcome to AUTEC," whispered Eli. "Atlantic Undersea Testing and Evaluation Center. Basically, it's the US Navy's not-so-secret installation for electronic warfare development and testing. I have an old friend stationed here that might be able to shed some light on the security situation in the area. I want to have a better idea of what to expect before we head out tomorrow."

"Well, you could have told me before we came down here," she said, somewhat indignantly.

"Like I've said before, sometimes things just happen in a certain way and you have to go with it. I saw the opportunity and here we are. Let's hope Perry can see us."

"Sir," called out the SP. "The Lieutenant Commander would like to speak with you."

The young guy held up the phone and Eli walked over to the guard shack. Both of the young SP's could not stop staring at Jo, who smiled back uncomfortably but held her ground.

"Yes, this is Eli Rose. Perry, you old SOB. How the hell have you been?"

"Bored out of my mind until you showed up," replied the voice on the phone.

"Can you meet us for dinner tonight? I need to talk to you."

"Us?" said Perry. "Who else is with you?"

"The girl I'm working for came along for the ride. So can I count on you?"

There was a pause on the other end of the line and then Perry answered, "Sure, what the hell. For an old friend like you, sure. Meet me at the Mangrove Bar at seven. But you owe me one from last time so you're buying."

"Deal," said Eli. "See you then."

"Wait," said Perry before Eli could hand over the receiver. "Put that SP back on."

Eli held the phone up to the SP. The kid listened for a few seconds and then said, "Aye, aye, sir. Right away," and hung up. "Daly, you're on watch until I get back. Sir, mam, if you please." The SP pointed at his jeep and it was clear that he intended for Eli and Jo to get in. They walked over and Eli got in the back, Jo in the front next to the kid.

"The Lieutenant Commander ordered me to drive you to the Mangrove Bar."

Jo raised her eyebrows and Eli smiled. The jeep sputtered to a start and the roared off towards town in a cloud of white dust.

Chapter 12

"Julio, I know what you say but I need your help," said Vicente in Spanish "This will be the thing that will get us back with our friends in Langley. You know what that will mean for all of us."

The silence on the other end of the phone was deafening for Vicente, but he persisted. "Look, my friend, This is a great chance to cause damage to Fidel and get some of this trash off our streets and away from our kids. What do you say?"

Julio had thought long and hard about what he would really do if Vicente ever called him for help, real help like what he was asking for now. He considered just hanging up on him, but in the end the opportunity was too good to pass up.

"You son of a bitch," he said, exasperated. "I tell you no help and the first thing you do is call me to ask for help. You are a real son of a bitch, you know that?"

"Yes, my friend, whatever you say. But will you help?"

"Yes, I'll make the contacts for you. I'll arrange for the work to be done and some of my guys to be on the dock waiting for them. You just be sure to call me the moment you know when they will arrive. I don't want any of my people taking unnecessary risks for these Colombian assholes. Understand?"

"Of course, whatever you want. When will you call me about the work?"

"I will let you know on Monday if we'll be ready. You can tell your new friend Paco we will be ready for his submarine when it arrives."

"Excellent, thank you very much. I won't forget this." Vicente was so relieved he almost dropped the telephone. "Goodbye."

Now he knew the plan could be accomplished. He had been terrified all day that he had over promised to Paco and could not deliver on the timetable he was given. It was tight, but Julio had a good network in Pinar del Río and he would get the work done.

Vicente knew the risks of not delivering on his deal with Paco, especially before he could set him up with the DEA. While he had no contacts with *that* agency, he did still have a couple of contacts at Langley he could call on for help. He needed to go to the office and have Rita call Jim Morgan. Morgan liked Rita, and likely he'd take her call even if she did pass him on to Vicente.

He drove down to the building and parked in his newly reserved space, locked the Corvette and started for the elevator. But his day, which had started with a delicate and stress-filled meeting with a major figure in the narcotics business, was about to get even more complicated.

Before he could take three steps from his car a large black Ford Econoline van roared up to him, seemingly from nowhere. The side door opened and two men wearing ski masks leaped out and shoved a pair of Glock Model 22's in Vicente's stomach and yelled, "Get in!" He instantly recognized the weapons as new FBI-issued firearms and complied without hesitation. They had moved to the Glocks after that disastrous shootout a few years before, when their standard issue .38 Specials couldn't put down those two bank robbers. If it had been any other circumstance, he would have disarmed the man on his right and used him as a shield against the one on his left. Fortunately, this wasn't necessary.

The two men sat beside him in the center seats while the driver and passenger sat silently in front. The van lurched from side to side as they exited the garage, twisting its way down Brickell Avenue. Vicente looked at the four men but each was still hidden by a ski mask. Their shoes were plain black wingtips and they each wore black trousers. One faux-gold Timex watch, one stainless steel Citizen chronograph; he couldn't see what the two men in front wore on their arms. It was all pretty conservative stuff, and reinforced his initial impression that the men were likely FBI, DEA, or from some other law enforcement agency.

"Would any of you gentlemen like to tell me why I am kidnap?" Vicente asked in his most polite and correct English. No one replied, so he continued.
"Can you tell me, where we go?" Still no reply.
"Can you tell me, you are FBI or DEA?"

This caused all four men to look at him, though the driver did so with only a glance in his mirror.

"Shut up," growled the passenger in the front. "You'll get your answers in a few minutes."

The van pulled into the parking garage of the Miami Center towers and the man on Vicente's right said, "Put this on - now!" He handed Vicente a black felt hood, so he put it on and sat calmly while the van came to a stop. The side door slid open with a bang and his guard said, "Move."

Vicente slid out of his seat carefully and felt a hand on his arm, guiding him down.

Once out of the van, his two companions each grabbed an elbow and escorted him to an elevator. The motion was not like that of a passenger elevator. *Must be a freight elevator,* he thought.

It took thirty seconds for the elevator to stop and twenty steps to reach the office they occupied, so Vicente thought he could probably find the floor and the office again if he needed to. He could hear computer keyboards being tapped and the muffled sounds of telephones ringing, but couldn't tell how many people were in the office. He was led through a door into a room with the air conditioning turned up too high, and one of the men yanked off his hood.

"Sit here," said one of the guys, pointing at a chair.

Vicente sat down and the four men left the room and closed the door. He took a minute to survey the setting. No windows, one door. One other chair, wood with a straight back. Light green paint on the walls, acoustic ceiling tiles; standard government issue. There was a pitcher of water on the table with two glasses, so he poured himself a glass and sat there quietly, knowing that someone was observing him through a hidden camera.

The door opened and a tall, middle-aged man in a black suit entered. He closed the door and sat down opposite Vicente, placing a manila folder on the table in front of him.

"I'm Special Agent Smith. I guess you want to know why you're here." He pulled his FBI identification and badge out quickly, allowing Vicente to confirm his identity.

"That would be very nice," said Vicente calmly. "I no realize that the FBI is in the business to kidnap people."

Smith frowned and open the folder, revealing several grainy photos of Vicente and Paco Gutiérrez, obviously taken from the bay and from a great distance.

"You know who this man is, so why don't you tell me what you were doing there?"

"This is a private business meeting," Vicente replied, staring directly into the agent's eyes. "Maybe you want to explain first what you are doing and why I here. Then maybe I talk with you."

The agent sat back in his chair and sighed. "It's not a crime just to do business with this guy. It just depends on what type of business you're doing, Mr.?"

"Amarón. Vicente Amarón."

Smith pulled a small note pad and a pen from his coat pocket and began writing. "What type of business are you in, Mr. Amarón?"

"I sorry, but I commit a crime? Do you arrest me now?"

"No, sir, you are not under arrest. At this point, all we want to do is ask you some questions."

"Well, before I give you some answer maybe you tell me what is this all about?"

Vicente was incredulous and was not going to give anything away. The agent obviously did not know who he was dealing with. *This guy will try to scare me into cooperating*, he thought. *If he knew who I was, maybe he would do this differently.* But he knew there was little chance of the FBI finding out about his background, since their database was thankfully not linked into the CIA database. So he sat there smiling confidently in his relative anonymity and happy for once at the inefficiency of government.

"Ok, fair enough. This is what I'll tell you, and if you ever want to get out of here you'll listen carefully and cooperate with us. This office is part of a joint FBI-DEA-ATF task force called named "Orchid." We are investigating the activities of your business partner, and we have reason to believe that Gutiérrez is the guy who was chosen by the Medellín Cartel to replace Carlos Lehder and Griselda Blanco to manage the import of cocaine into Miami. We think he is also responsible for bringing in several shipments of illegal weapons from Cuba and has plans to continue all of this. We consider anyone who goes to a meeting at his place to be a person of interest, because Gutiérrez doesn't allow just anyone to have access to him. So Mr. Amarón, what I want to know is, what type of business are you in and just what did you discuss with Paco Gutiérrez?"

The agent returned the stare and now Vicente knew he'd have to say something. He hadn't prepared for this situation, hadn't concocted a cover for his cover, so the truth seemed like the best option. Or maybe just part of the truth.

"Special Agent Smith, thank you for tell me why I here. For my part, I work for Brickell Avenue Associates and we make an investigation into the disappearance of two very rich people. I think this guy Gutiérrez is involve in this, so I try to get close to him to find out what happen. To do this I facilitate a shipment of cocaine from Colombia to Mexico. I was plan to alert the authorities about this before the shipment arrive."

"Yes, I'm sure you were," said Smith sarcastically. "So is this plan moving forward or did he tell you to go away?"

"The plan move forward right now. I call him next Wednesday to arrange a meeting to confirm the detail and then is up to him."

Smith scribbled some notes and said, "Ok, Mr. Amarón. Here's what we can offer you. In return for your cooperation with this investigation, you will have immunity from prosecution. But you have to cooperate fully with us. Understand?"

It was not the first time Vicente had been offered such a deal from the US government. He'd successfully avoided this type of thing for more than five years but through no fault of his own, was stuck once again with having to make a tough choice.

"Of course I will help you in whatever way I can," he said with a smile.

At that moment another agent entered, handed Smith a note and left immediately without speaking.

"Good," said Smith, looking at the note. "We'll be sending a team by your apartment this afternoon to tap your phone. We'll also put a radio-frequency identification device, an RFID, in your car so we can track you if we need to. Just be sure to keep us informed of everything you're planning and this will work out just fine. Are we clear about this?"

"Very clear. I can go now?"

"Yes. Wait here a moment." Smith shuffled his photos back into the folder and left the room. A moment later, two agents wearing ski masks and holding the black hood entered the room.

"You know the drill," said the agent with the hood. He extended it to Vicente, who put it on and was led from the room.

They walked back out of the office and twenty steps over to the elevator. After the thirty second trip they were soon back in the van and driving toward Brickell Avenue Associates. The hood was removed as the van pulled up outside the building.

"Have a nice day," said one of his escorts. The other men laughed while the guy on his right opened the side door.

"Thank you," said Vicente. "And the same for you." He went into the lobby and took the elevator to the office.

"Well, look at what the cat dragged in," said Rita.

"Good morning to you also," he replied. "Have you receive any call from Eli?"

"Nothing yet. Why, are you expecting something?"

Vicente shook his head and went to his office. Rita

followed him in and he started writing some notes on his pad.

"If he call in I want you to tell him this: I am in with Paco Gutiérrez and that part move Ok, but the FBI is watch everything I do. Is all here so you no forget."

"I won't forget. So what's up? How did you get tied up with the FBI?"

Vicente groaned and rolled his eyes at the ceiling. "Is no important so don worry. But I want you to tell me if you have a visit from a person you don know. If that happen you must go to visit you sister in Orlando for a couple of weeks. Understand?" He looked at her with all the seriousness he could project, and she got the message very clearly.

"Vicente, this doesn't sound good. Maybe we should call Jim Morgan. He can maybe help or know someone we can call." She smacked her gum nervously and was obviously worried. "I don't want nothin' to happen to you guys."

He smiled and patted her on the arm. "You no worry about me and Eli. We know how to take care of ourself. But if someone come here to ask question you must tell me and then leave town."

"Ok," she answered hesitantly. "I got it." She picked up Vicente's notes and walked back to her desk. "You sure about this?"

"Yes, I am certain."

He sat back for a moment and contemplated the situation. He could play things out with the FBI, risking exposure and a very bad fate at the hands of Paco Gutiérrez, or he could call Morgan and appeal to him for help. *I think I will keep Morgan in my back pocket until I need him*, he thought. *It is already complicated enough.*

Rita brought him a *cafecito* and he propped his feet up on his desk. *I bet Eli is having a good trip with this girl. Always he has the easy part.* Vicente smiled to himself and tossed back the small black coffee in one gulp.

§

"I'm starving," said Jo as she glanced at the plastic-coated menu. "What's good here?"

"I have no idea," Eli replied, "but I'd stick to whatever fish is local if I was you."

The waiter came over and delivered two large glasses of water while they waited for Perry Barnes to arrive. He was late but Eli was not surprised. His schedule could be unpredictable because of his involvement in the monitoring exercises that were conducted at AUTEC, and Eli suspected they were in the middle of one when he and Jo showed up at the gate. Just at that moment, Perry came in the open entrance, wearing a colorful Hawaiian-style shirt and khaki trousers.

"Wow, the Navy is getting pretty casual these days," exclaimed Eli as he embraced his friend.

"Yeah, don't I wish," said Perry. "I'm off duty this weekend so I can dress down a little tonight. And you are?" He turned to Jo, shaking her hand.

"Jo McHenry. Good to meet you, Perry."

"The pleasure's mine," he answered, winking at Eli.

"If I'd known that this guy was in the company of such a beautiful woman I'd have been early."

"Have a seat," said Eli. "So how is business these days?"

"Oh, you know, same old stuff. Just plodding along, doing what we do, making the world a safer place." The waiter returned to the table and Perry said, "Bring me a cold Kalik, would you?"

"Yes, sir," said the waiter.

"So what brings you two to this paradise?"

Eli had decided long ago that only option with Perry Barnes was to be completely open and honest or he would get stonewalled.

"Perry, Jo's parents have gone missing on a sailing holiday. They may have passed through here about a month ago, but they haven't checked in and they haven't been seen by anyone. I talked with Leslie in Nassau and none of his people have heard anything. I was hoping you could pass along some "unofficial" intel on what's been going on around these parts lately."

The waiter brought his beer and Perry said, "Let's order something," side-stepping the request. "Jo, I'm sure you're hungry after that long trip. Why don't you start?"

Jo ordered the grilled grouper, and the others followed suit. They sat there silently until the waiter went back to the kitchen and then Perry leaned in close.

"Look Eli, this kind of stuff is strictly off the record, as usual. Just rumors, shit we hear sometimes when we are running an exercise." He looked around to make sure no one was listening and continued.

"We've had some trouble out here lately with pirates

and drug runners. We've had to send our testing vessels out with an armed escort on a few occasions because of some chatter we picked up around Norman's Cay."

"Norman's Cay? I thought that was shut down years ago by the RBDF?" said Eli with surprise.

"What's Norman's Cay?" asked Jo.

"Norman's Cay," said Perry, "is where Carlos Lehder and the Medellín Cartel used to stage their cocaine shipments before entry into Miami. They'd fly them in using Max Mermelstein's guys and it worked well until Lehder got too public. These are pretty remote islands, and with all the comings and goings it attracted too much attention." He took a big drink of the beer and added, "About two months ago we started hearing the same kind of chatter over there that we'd picked up in the late '70's. We thought the place might be active again so we tipped the Bahamians. They went over there last week and found a bunch of dead Jamaicans, and no one knew who they were. The official word was that they were migrants who had come over looking for jobs but died of exposure on the trip. Rumor has it they were shot up pretty badly."

"You don't think they were just looking for jobs, do you Perry?" Eli knew that his friend had most of the story figured out.

"Not at all," he said. The food arrived and they all paused to take a few bites, enjoying the sweet fish and relaxing in the light evening breeze.

"The Jamaicans," Perry continued, "They were almost certainly Shower Posse guys. But why they were hanging out there is a mystery. Anyway, a few weeks ago a group of Cuban guys show up in three big

Donzi's. According to the guys at the ferry terminal, they came in, fueled up and went back out without talking to anyone. Not something you see every day here, so once again, some strange stuff going on. And when did you last hear from your parents?"

"A little more than three weeks ago when they headed out," said Jo through a mouthful of fish. "But they should have been back more than a week ago. That's when I contacted Eli for help."

Eli had already pieced together a scenario that explained almost everything, but he wasn't about to tell anyone just yet. "So that's it? Nothing else out of the ordinary?"

"Nope," said Perry. "Just you and your beautiful boss here."

Jo smiled. Eli changed the subject and they began to talk about Miami, the state of the economy, and a variety of less stressful but mildly interesting topics. After an hour the waiter arrived with the check and Eli pulled thirty Bahamian dollars from his wallet and put them on the table.

"Perry, we're going to take off now. We've got an early morning and a lot to do before we head back to Nassau."

They got up from the table and Eli gave his friend a hug again. "I owe you for the information," he said. Eli held onto Perry as he was about to pull away and whispered into his ear, "Listen, we're due back in Nassau on Monday. Do me a favor and call Leslie by Monday night. If we haven't checked in with him, call out the cavalry."

Perry held his friend at arm's length for a moment to

see if he was joking. When he saw that Eli was serious, he said, "Sure, pal. I won't let you down. Er, goodnight, Jo. It was great meeting you. I hope you find your parents real soon."

"Thanks Perry. It was my pleasure."

Jo turned to leave and Perry said to Eli, "Hey, bro, if you think you're going to be in some kind of trouble, you shouldn't go out tomorrow."

"Thanks man," said Eli, "but I've got to get to the bottom of this. Just do me a favor and watch my back."

"You bet." The two men embraced again and went their separate ways.

Eli and Jo untied the little raft and motored back to the *Bree-zee*. Neither one spoke on the way back until they reached the swimming ladder. Jo tied them off and then they both clambered onto the deck. "We can bring the raft up tomorrow before we leave," said Eli. They went below decks and locked the cabin door.

Jo went in to use the marine head while Eli fixed up the bunk. It was warm but the wind sock provided a small breeze to help ventilate the cabin. Jo came out of the head completely nude and Eli was again dumbstruck by her body. She lifted the mosquito net and joined him at the bunk. She gave him a hug and then kissed him, exploring his mouth with her tongue. He kissed her back and she pressed up against him.

"Is that a banana in your pocket or are you just happy to see me?" Jo said with a laugh. She reached into his shorts and was happily rewarded. "Oh, so you're happy to see me. That's good."

Jo worked her magic again and they made love slowly in the dimly lit cabin, taking time to experiment and learn more about each other's bodies. In the end, she laid beside him and said, "Do you think we'll ever find them?"

"I don't know, maybe," answered Eli, though he suspected otherwise. Donald and Madeleine McHenry were gone, most likely murdered. He was certain of that much. What he didn't know was why.

Chapter 13

"Are you ready?" Eli called out.

"Yes, ready when you are," yelled Jo. She motored up slowly on the anchor line and Eli broke it loose, winching it up and locking it down quickly. Jo turned the wheel hard to the right and they slipped out into the middle of Fresh Creek, headed back out of Andros Town.

They had awakened early when a brief thunderstorm passed over the town, spraying water in on them from the open hatch. It was good timing though, since first light came shortly after, so they were able to get going before seven. Eli sat and reviewed the map with her before they started, but kept the map and the binoculars at the ready. He'd also stowed his Beretta and the L85 in the line locker so he could get to them quickly if he needed to.

Jo steered the boat out while Eli uncleated the sails. It would take them about six and a half hours to get to the Joulters Cays, and he wanted to have plenty of light at a high angle so he could spot the sand bars and patch reefs easily. Once they'd cleared the mouth of the channel, Eli raised the main and mizzen and Jo, as always, hoisted the Genoa.

"Ok, boss, you're on," said Eli, and Jo turned northwest. "You can see the drop off, so just stay right at the edge and we'll be fine."

She nodded and sat back against the cushion. The east wind helped them gain speed quickly, but that benefit was offset by the beam seas they would have to endure all the way there. Eli grabbed the fishing poles and set them up at the aft rail with large tuna lures. They needed to looked the part of tourists for any curious passersby, and they might even catch something for dinner that night.

Eli took over after two hours and they sailed a straight course of three thirty five degrees, paralleling the island. One of the rods suddenly screamed out and Jo jumped up to grab it, pulling back hard. Eli turned east to dump wind from the sails and suddenly Jo was into a fight with whatever was on the other end of the line.

"Eli, I don't think I can do this," she said, straining to hold the pole.

"Sure you can," he said with a smile. "If he runs just let him run. When he's quiet like this you need to pull up on the pole and reel in fast. Yep, just like that. Keep going. Pull up and reel in, pull up and reel in."

"My arms are killing me," she said.

"Ok, hang on," said Eli. He put a bungee cord around the wheel so it would stay roughly pointed east, and he jumped in next to her, wrapping his arms around her and grabbing the pole.

"Now we both pull. Ready - pull. Reel. Pull. Reel.

There we go, he's coming."

The fish finally surfaced close to the boat and Eli said, "It's a small black fin tuna. Hang on, don't lose him. We'll eat good tonight if we can bring him in."

Jo struggled to hang onto the pole but finally the fish was next to the boat. Eli grabbed a gaff hook and flipped the fish onto the deck. It flopped and jumped wildly, but Jo had her fish.

"Congratulations," Eli yelled. He gave Jo a big hug and she hugged him back.

"My arms feel like they're going to fall off," she gasped. She handed Eli the poll and said, "Ok, I caught him. Now it's your problem."

Eli laughed and unhooked the fish. He reset the pole while Jo unlocked the wheel, and they continued north along the drop off. Eli grabbed the fish and threw it in one of the large coolers below decks. He came back with two bottles of water, which Jo downed rapidly. He washed the blood off the deck and then grabbed the wheel.

"Why don't you take a break. I'll take her north from here."

"That was hard work," she exclaimed. "I *need* a break." She leaned her head against his shoulder and stretched out on the cushion, and she was asleep in less than a minute.

The sun beat down on the Bimini top and baked the deck, but the breeze created by their passage kept Eli and Jo cool and refreshed. The boat rocked gently in the beam swells and Eli concentrated on trying to flatten out the ride as much as possible, hoping the girl would sleep for a couple more hours. The best thing for her would be to get as much rest as possible, since he didn't know what lay before them.

Anyway, he needed some quiet time to think. The last twenty four hours had given him a lot to consider, especially since this girl, who had been so adversarial earlier in their relationship, was now as cooperative and compassionate as a long-time lover. The night before he left, Eli heard about her relationship with Lloyd Taylor from Vicente. That seemed more in character with the early version of Jo McHenry, the spoiled, self-centered one. It made perfect sense to Eli that she would use any means at her disposal to achieve her ends, including using her obvious charms to manipulate people to get what she wanted. And according to Vicente, what she seemed to want most was time.

Was any of what happened between us real? thought Eli. *Only partly*, he guessed. She definitely enjoyed herself but he was certain she was trying to gain his confidence, his unwavering loyalty. *Remember*, he said to himself, *she said she could wrap any man around her little finger, and I guess that includes me. She's paying me a million bucks to find her parents. Why bother with the rest?* He couldn't answer that last question yet. He was also sure she would want him to keep quiet about everything as well. Her father's involvement with a major illegal narcotics figure, her own cocaine addiction, probably more. *She must be sneaking a blow when she's below decks*, he thought.

Having all these ugly things become public would definitely ruin her chances to run her father's business empire. Eli decided he would continue to play along.

He needed to know what else was at stake, and how far she might want him to go once they'd gotten to the bottom of her parents disappearance.

He was getting stiff after two and a half hours and finally had to stand and straighten out his back and legs. Jo woke up and looked around for a second as if disoriented, then rolled over on her stomach and stretched out her arms.

"Oh, that was very nice," she said, smiling. "I really needed that. How are you doing?"

"A little stiff but Ok. If you look off there to the west you can see Nicholls Town."

She grabbed the binoculars and stared past him. "Yes, I see. Does that mean we're getting close?"

"Pretty close," he said. "About an hour and a half before we get there. Why don't you drive for awhile? I'm going to butcher the tuna so we can have it for a couple of days."

"Sure," she said, swinging her long legs under the wheel.

Eli went below and grabbed the tuna, his knife, and a few Ziploc bags and went back to the aft deck, where he proceeded to cut large filets from the tuna. He placed each one in a separate bag and then tossed the carcass off the back. The filets were put on ice and then he cleaned the deck before going back below. All the domestic work also gave him an opportunity to search Jo's bag for the cocaine he suspected was there, but after a brief look in the obvious places, he wasn't able to locate the contraband. *The stuff must be hidden around here somewhere*, he thought. But he couldn't find anything, and now he needed to go back on deck and start watching the water for their approach to the Joulters.

Eli stood on deck to get a better angle to view the water ahead and as they drew closer Jo yelled out, "I can see some trees."

It was the larger island of South Joulters, and they advanced from the south until Eli could clearly see the beach on the east side. "Jo, put her dead on. I want to go in with the motor only."

She turned the *Bree-zee* east towards the deep blue water and Eli lowered the mainsail and cranked in the Genoa. He lowered and secured the mizzen and then Jo turned back towards the beach. The boat bobbed and weaved as it was pushed from behind by the swells.

"Just go straight in there, away from the tidal channel and I'll tell you when to stop," he called out. Eli scanned the water ahead and finally waved at Jo.

"Turn her east and then we'll drift in and let the anchor hook us up." He was a little nervous about doing that, since the coarse lime sands of the bottom around South Joulters didn't offer much for the anchor to hook up on, but that was a reasonable first choice.

Jo headed east and at Eli's signal, put the engine in neutral. He dropped the large anchor and waited for what seemed like an eternity while the *Bree-zee* bobbed and drifted towards the beach.

"Eli," Jo called out nervously, looking back at the rapidly approaching sand.

"Just a minute," he answered, watching the anchor line.

"Eli, we're getting too close."

"There, she's hooked," he exclaimed with relief. "I'll go in and check the anchor and make sure we're in good. Hang the safety line and float off the back."

He grabbed a mask, fins, and snorkel from the storage locker and went over the side towards the anchor line. Looking down from the surface, Eli could see that the anchor was hooked under a small coral head on the sandy bottom. He took a couple of deep breaths and kicked up, diving down to check the security of the anchor. He pulled himself down and then put his feet on either side of the flukes, pulling up on the line. It held tight and he pushed off to get a breath at the surface.

He swam back to the safety line and pulled himself back to the swim ladder. "Jo?" he called up. There was no answer. "Jo?" he yelled more loudly this time. Still no answer. He pulled off his fins and climbed back up on deck. Just as he was about to go look for her in the cabin she appeared with a towel and a bottle of water.

"I thought you might need these," she said, tossing him the towel.

"Thanks. I'm going to put out a spring line for the tide change, so I'll be back in a minute."

He cleated off a second anchor line and threw the smaller spare Danforth over the side. Eli dove down and picked the anchor up and carried it back to their starboard side, jabbing the flukes tightly into the sand. He swam back and stripped off the mask and snorkel and dried himself off.

"We won't drift now," he said to Jo. "We can space out the watches a bit more, say every four hours now."

"That's good," she replied. "I'm still pretty tired,

even after my nap this morning." She smiled and sat down.

"So, what's the plan now?"

"Well," said Eli, "the plan is to fire up the oven and have a late lunch or early dinner, and plan tomorrow's search before we lose our light."

"Ok, how can I help?"

"Can you cut up some vegetables for me?" said Eli.

Jo looked surprised. "Well, I'm not much for cooking, but I can make a really good boat drink."

"That's fine," said Eli. *Not surprising at all that she can't even cut up a vegetable*, he thought.

"Sure, make some good boat drinks and that will work great."

He went below to start cutting up some vegetables to roast with the tuna. Jo set up her supplies on the other side of the galley and began what looked like a serious chemistry experiment, mixing and blending a variety of canned fruit juices with several different rums that Eli had requested for the ship's stores. He slipped the roasting pan into the oven just as she completed her first blend of drinks.

"I call this one "Jo's Jam," she said with a smile, handing him a glass. "What do you think?"

Eli took a sip and shook his head. "Wow." It was super strong and very sweet, but tasty. "That's really good," he said. "But really strong. You might consider lightening up on the rum for the next round."

"Why would I want to do something like that? Besides, maybe I'll just get you drunk and then take advantage of you." She smiled salaciously and flicked her tongue across the rim of her glass.

"Sounds great to me, but not until later. We need to go over the maps and the plan for tomorrow first."

She chugged down her drink and started working on another mix. "This one will be better," she said.

Eli went into his bag for the other maps he needed while Jo experimented with her dangerous brew. He put a map of Andros Island and the Joulters Cays on the galley table and said, "Since you're so intent on getting us both drunk I think we better look at this now."

She suddenly exclaimed, "That's the one! You'll like this one."

Eli was trying not to become frustrated with the girl, but her attitude wasn't helpful. He was still trying to do a job, no matter how much she seemed to be enjoying it. "Can we focus over here for a minute?"

"Oh, well, don't get you're panties in a wad," she said. "I thought we were having fun, and then you go and get all serious."

"Jo, you're paying me a lot of money to find out what happened to your parents, and you deserve to have all of my attention while we're out here. I'm not trying to be a hardass, but from my perspective I have a job to do. Do you understand?"

She frowned and pouted for a second. "Sure, I get it." She moved in closer to look at the map.

"Here, take this one. It's better than the first one. Show me what you're planning."

Eli took a sip of the drink, decidedly much better than the first one, and put it down.

"We're here, just off the southern tip of South Joulters. If your parents came ashore they may have left some sign that they were here. In the morning we'll take the raft and land here. We can look through the island for an hour or so and then we'll take off and head up to north Joulters and see if we can find anything there. After that, we can go on up to the Berry's and see if they stopped in there. Heck, we may even find them there, anchored out and sipping boat drinks."

Jo put her drink down and looked closely at the map. She was no more than an inch from his face, and he caught the strong smell of rum on her breath.

"That sounds like a good plan," she said turning so that their lips almost touched. "Do you really think we'll ever find them?"

She kept asking him the same question and it was still a tough question to answer honestly. He didn't want her to lose hope, yet every ounce of his intuition and experience told him that her parents were dead and would never be found.

"Maybe, Jo. I don't know. I want to believe we can still turn up something, some clue or maybe even find the boat somewhere. But honestly, I don't know."

She sat back against the seat cushion and began to tear up. "It's my fault they did this," she said, sobbing. "It's my fault they're lost. I should have gone with them. I told Father that I was too busy to go this time. I said I had my own life and that he couldn't expect me to go with him anymore. If I'd have gone, maybe I could have helped or done something." She began to cry and Eli put his arm around her shoulder and hugged her.

"Come on, Jo. You know that if you'd have gone you would be missing, too. There's nothing you could have done to prevent this. It's not your fault." She cried into his chest, maybe the first good cry she'd had since the whole affair started.

"You don't understand," she said softly. "We had a fight the week before, a really bad fight. Father had promised me that he would get me voted onto the Board of Directors, and that when he retired next year that I would take his place as CEO. I pressed him about it and he said he'd had a change of heart, that I wasn't ready and that Lloyd should take over. That was the last time we spoke. I never wanted this. I never wanted things to end up like this."

She cried again and Eli did his best to comfort her. He felt conflicted about her, knowing what he knew, but her sadness seemed genuine. He held her face up and said, "We'll get an answer. We'll find out what happened, I promise you." She nodded and he said, "Let's get something to eat. You'll feel better and then we can finish our planning for tomorrow."

Eli turned off the oven and put the steaming pan of fish on the range. "Come and get a plate." He served her a large piece of the broiled tuna and vegetables and they ate quickly.

"It's really good," she said. "Where did you learn this?"

"Just picked it up over the years. I'm glad you like it."

"It's yummy." She was quiet for a moment and then said, "You know, you haven't told me very much about yourself. All I really know is what I picked up here and there from other people."

"Well, there's not much to tell," Eli replied. He wasn't interested in having to side-step through his life story, but it seemed inevitable that he'd have to answer some questions.

"Oh, I see," she said between bites. "One thing I don't know is, have you ever been married? Was there ever a Mrs. Rose, or have you always been a devoted bachelor?"

'The only Mrs. Rose there has ever been was my mother," he answered. "There were a couple of women here and there that meant something, but one thing led to another and things didn't work out."

Jo reflected on his answer and said, "So does that mean you have commitment issues, or you just like "playing the field?"

Eli smiled and shook his head. "In my line of work it's a good thing to have commitment issues. And I don't really have much time to "play the field." Jo sat silently after his answer and finished her fish.

He collected the plates and rinsed them in the ocean, tossing the uneaten portions into the water.

"Let's finish this so we can hit the sack. Tomorrow, we'll wait until about nine before we go ashore so we can see everything clearly. Take some long pants, your rain jacket, and your tennis shoes. There are a lot of thorns and sharp scrub on that island and you'll need something to cover your legs or you'll get chewed up. Plus, the deer flies are pretty ferocious, so the more clothes the better. We'll take some water and our ditch bag, just in case we have to send off a signal. And these." Eli reached over and opened the galley locker where he kept his Beretta and the L85 light machine gun.

"Oh my God!" she said. "What are you doing with those guns? Do you seriously think we'll need those?"

He sighed. "I hope we don't, but I'd rather have them if I need them then not have them." He handed her the Beretta. "Do you know how to use one of these?"

She held it gingerly and not too securely by the handle. "You don't get much practice with guns in the fashion industry," she said, forcing a smile.

He took the pistol back and said, "Ok, watch carefully. This lever here - this is the safety. Make sure you click it like this to turn the safety off. Then you pull back on the slide - see the grips on the sides. That chambers a round. Then it's point and shoot. You have fifteen rounds per clip, and I have five extra clips, so you shouldn't need all of them. When you fire, keep both eyes open and look straight down the barrel through the front sites. It's only for close range self defense, so let's hope you don't ever have to use it."

"Yeah, for sure," she said.

It was getting dark and the seas and breeze began to die down. Eli said, "I'll stand the first watch if you want to get some sleep."

"That's Ok. Do you mind if I stay up with you for a little while?"

"No, that would be great," he replied.

Eli put the weapons out on the table and assembled the rest of the gear he needed in the ditch bag, then went out onto the deck with the binoculars. The sun was setting behind the island and Jo soon appeared in her rain jacket and took a seat beside him.

"It's so peaceful here," she said. "No rat race, no complications, only you and the sea. I wish everything could be this simple." She hugged his arm and put her head on his shoulder.

"Nothing is ever this simple," Eli answered.

"You know, Eli, I really like you. You're different. You're not like any of the other men I've known." She hugged him tightly. "I know that I'm paying you to do a job, but I feel a closer connection to you than that. Can you tell me how you feel?"

It was a tough question, because he couldn't win regardless of how he answered. If he answered in the negative, she would be sad and might become hostile and uncooperative again. If he answered in the positive, she might believe she'd won him over and was in complete control of him.

"I like you a lot, too. You are really unpredictable, but you're also very exciting to be with and full of life. You energize me like no one ever has."

She smiled and took his hand, kissing his palm. "I'm glad. That makes me happy." She moved his hand to her breast and said, "So maybe you could perform another service as part of your job."

He began to stroke her softly and they kissed. The sun reflected in shades of orange and pink off the high clouds and bathed them in a warm glow. She repositioned his hand between her upper thighs and opened her legs. "You know what to do," she sighed.

He kissed her neck and her back while he massaged her, drawing gasps and low moans from her until he'd worked her to the brink of climax.

"Don't stop," she panted. She laid back against his chest and he helped her finish. She grabbed his hand and pressed it deep into her until she relaxed and her breathing slowed down closer to normal.

"Now it's your turn," she said with a smile.

Chapter 14

"Eli, wake up." He heard the whisper but didn't immediately recognize the voice. "Eli, Eli. Are you awake?"

"Yeah, I'm up." He threw his feet over the bunk and sat up, dazed but aware that Jo was kneeling next to him. He looked at his watch. Four in the morning. Too early for him to relieve her on watch. He'd just gone to sleep two hours before. "What's up?"

"Eli, I think I heard something," she whispered.

"Heard something where?"

"Out there, down to the south. It sounded like a really big engine but it was pretty far away."

"Ok, let me see." They went on deck quietly and Eli took the binoculars from her. He scanned the horizon and then the island but could see nothing.

"We'll, whatever it was it's gone now. If it's a problem, we'll know in the morning. You go below and get some rest. I'll finish the watch."

"Are you sure?"

"Yeah, go ahead."

The girl went below and Eli settled in on deck with

the binoculars. It was a brilliant, starring night, and there was enough residual light to be able to see the beach and first line of Australian pines on the dunes just behind it, but not much more. He settled back against the rear cushion, listening for anything other than the sound of the wind cutting through the rigging and the waves lapping rhythmically against the hull. Nothing. Maybe she'd just imagined it? He didn't know, but caution was the best course of action until they could investigate the island after dawn.

Eli must have dozed for a few minutes because he was awakened by the first rays of the new morning sun on his unshaven face. It warmed him quickly so he went below to grab a bottle of water and some crackers for breakfast. Jo was still sleeping so he came back up on deck to launch the raft. After some effort he was able to slide off the side and tie it to the swim ladder. The wind was light and the seas were mostly calm, so Eli thought they would be able to use the tidal channel to get behind the island. The tide was going in as well, and that would help.

Jo appeared at the cabin door and asked, " When do you want to get moving?" She rubbed her eyes and face, waking slowly.

"Maybe a half hour or so. If we don't find anything quickly we should start moving north. That will take awhile so we better get going soon."

He went back to the cabin and loaded the rest of his supplies into the ditch bag: water, flares, a mirror, matches, medical supplies, the binoculars, his hat and long sleeved fishing shirt, the Beretta and the L85. He stripped in front of Jo, who looked on with a smile, then put on his khaki's and tennis shoes. Jo did the same but wore a white top without a bra, reminding Eli how strikingly attractive she was. She put on her floppy hat and went up on deck.

"After you," said Eli, and Jo climbed down onto the raft. He handed her the heavy ditch bag and climbed in. He choked the little motor and pulled the cord and it started again on the first try. "I'll drive, so you need to untie us."

Jo freed them from the line and left it in the water so they could pick it up easily when they returned. Eli turned the raft to his right and headed for the tidal channel to his south. The tide was moving in and the current ran fast through the channel, so he turned into a small creek just at the end of the tree-covered dunes. He'd motored slowly up the creek for only a few seconds when he saw something very disturbing. Just ahead and slightly to his left was some debris that had washed onto the mud flat, mostly likely at high tide. He steered over to get as close as possible and then beached the nose of the raft on the flats.

"You stay here with your hand on the tiller," Eli said. "I'm going to see what that is over there."

They switched places and he took off his pants, shoes and socks and jumped over the side. The water was only shin deep but the mud on the flats was hot and sulfidic. He sunk in up to his knees, making walking nearly impossible. He struggled on through the mud, trying to ignore the stinging irritation on his skin. Finally, he reached the edge of the debris field and had a chance to examine the pieces.

The first couple of things he looked over were non-descript pieces of plastic. As he sifted through the small pile he found a couple of seat cushions.

"Do you remember the color of the seat cushions on your parents boat?" Eli called over to Jo.

"They were kind of silvery-gray on white I think," she answered. "Why? Have you found something?"

Uh-oh. That's not good, he thought. That was the color pattern of the cushion he was holding.

"Nothing yet," he lied.

He needed more than a seat cushion to understand what happened, so he slogged on through the sticky mud for another few yards and reached another small pile of debris. This one had some rigging and lines twisted into it, again with nothing too promising. Then he saw it. It was lying under a section of plastic decking and Eli's stomach knotted up when he recognized what it was. He struggled over and pulled out the life preserver ring. When he flipped it over he saw what he feared most. The name was clearly visible - *Madeleine*. He pulled on the decking and saw what looked like several large caliber bullet holes in it. A bucket, some other fragments of plastic, and then a shoe, stained dark red. He needed no other evidence.

Eli replaced the shoe under the debris pile but held the life ring and carried it back through the mud. He washed off the mud before he got back into the raft and then handed the ring to Jo. She immediately began to cry.

"Eli, they're dead, they're dead. I knew it. Oh, God Eli." She cried hard and he tried to comfort her as best he could.

"We still don't know for sure," he said, though he felt certain that it was true. "Maybe they're on the island somewhere and injured. Or they couldn't salvage anything to make a signal fire. We still need to check the island, just to be sure they aren't out there, somewhere."

Jo sobbed and looked up at him, nodding her head. Tears streamed down her cheeks and she struggled to regain control. "Ok, if you think so."

"Jo, it looks really bad, and I don't want you to think there's much hope. But we've got to check it out."

She nodded again so Eli put his pants and shoes back on and pushed back off the mud flat. The tide had just started going out so he rode the current around to the front of the island and landed the raft on a wide stretch of beach. They got out and Eli pulled the raft up to the rock line and tied the bow ring to a tree. He pulled the ditch bag over his shoulder and said, "Follow me."

Eli had been on the island when he was much younger. *El Grupo* had used it as a training base when their Everglades firing range was discovered by the police. It was a longer trip for them, but since the islands are uninhabited, they were able to stage live-firing exercises without much fear of interruption. It was little changed from what he remembered; low, scrub bushes and shrubs in the interior, a mix of bright white sand and grey rocky dunes, and small salt pans and saline ponds. There was no cover to speak of, and the deer flies found them as soon as they cleared the beach. Their long clothes helped fend off the vicious insects and protected them from the thorny bushes while they trudged inland.

"There's a high dune over there and we should be able to see pretty much everything here from that vantage point."

Eli led the way and they climbed the ridge. He used the binoculars to scan the interior of the island but saw nothing. However, not far from where they had first landed he saw another debris pile, this one ominously larger than the first.

"I think there's not much down here," he said, handing her a bottle of water.

Jo sat down and drank silently, hanging her head so as not to look at him. Tears still streamed down her face and Eli sat down beside her with his arms around her shoulders.

"I was so mean to them the last time I saw them," she said hoarsely. "I took them for granted, like they'd always be around and now I've lost them. I was so stupid."

"I know how you feel," he said. "I felt the same way when my parents passed. It's hard to deal with, because nothing anyone can say will ever make you feel differently. You just have to move past it and go on."

She looked at him and nodded. "It just hurts so..........."

"Hold on," he interrupted.

"I know, I'm just going on and on. I should.............."

"No, it's not you," he said in a lowered voice. "Listen." They sat there quietly for a second and suddenly she could hear it, too. Voices. Two or three men, and it sounded like Spanish.

"Eli, what are we going to do?" she whispered.

He tore into the ditch bag and pulled out the weapons.

"You take this," he said, handing her the Beretta. "Move over there, near that bush, and stay down."

She grasped the pistol and flipped off the safety, then scrambled quickly in behind the bush. Eli clicked off the safety on the L85 and pulled the bolt back slowly. He stayed low but peered over the dune as the talking became louder and more clear.

They sounded like Cubans! *Oh shit*, he thought. *They're looking for the drugs.* There were three of them, and they were armed with MAC-10's equipped with large suppressors, and that meant that Eli was out-gunned. They stopped at the top of a nearby dune and the increased conversation told Eli that their raft had been seen. One of the guys pulled a radio from his pocket and said, "Donzi, Donzi, come in. We found a raft and we think they are on the island. We need some help here."

"We are coming," was the barely distinct answer.

Eli could hear the roar of large engines in the distance and he realized that they would soon be running for their lives. Their only hope would be to steal one of the boats when the men landed on the island. They were coming in fast so Eli motioned for Jo to move back to their right, down the dunes to the south. The three Cubans stood there talking quietly while one of them lit a cigarette. Jo and Eli moved along the back side of the high dune and were out of view until they reached the end of the dune. They had to cover a small expanse of open ground before they could reach the safety of the tree line, and unfortunately, they would have to risk exposing themselves to get across it.

"Ok, we're going to have to run," he whispered. "I'll go across first and then I'll cover you. On a count of three. Ready - one, two, three."

He sprinted across the space, maybe twenty yards and managed to make the trees without being noticed. He waved at Jo and she nodded. She jumped up and started running but tripped on a large rock and fell loudly, flat on her stomach.

"Hey, did you see that?" yelled one of the men. "It's them!" He squeezed of a short burst from his MAC-10 and the .45 ACP rounds ricocheted around in all directions.

Jo got up and ran the rest of the way to Eli, prompting the others to fire. Eli retuned fire with the L85 and the three men dove for cover. Eli was desperate. He knew they were in a bad situation with few options, and likely they couldn't fight their way out of the mess they were in. The two Donzi's must have reached the beach because he heard their loud engines suddenly cut off, accompanied by the sound of more voices getting closer.

Shot were fired into the trees around them and Eli motioned for Jo to back down closer to the beach. Their backs were to the water and there was little more they could do. He fired another burst into the dunes close to the largest group of men and they crouched for cover again.

"Give me this," he said, grabbing the Beretta from Jo. He wrapped it in a handkerchief and shoved it under a fallen tree. Then he called out in Spanish, "Ok, we give up. No more shooting, we give up."

Eli reached back and threw the L85 towards the dunes, and the men rushed in, weapons drawn. They quickly encircled the pair and pulled them to their feet. There were six young guys, maybe in their early twenties and one older guy in his thirties, and they were all filthy and stunk of sweat and mud. They all had long black hair and wore white shirts, but with green camouflage pants and jungle boots. *Definitely not locals*, thought Eli.

The oldest guy approached him and said, "So who are you assholes and what are you doing here?"

"We're tourists," said Eli, knowing what the reaction would be. "We just stopped here over night and we're doing some exploring."

"Exploring?" said the older guy. He shoved his gun hard into Eli's stomach, causing him to bend forward in pain. The guy grabbed Eli by the shirt and added, "With a gun like the one you just used? You want to tell me again what you're doing here?"

"Ok, Ok. We're looking for the drugs."

The guy let Eli go and went over to confer with another one of the group. Jo held Eli's hand and said, "What's going on? Who are they?"

"Narco-traffickers," whispered Eli. "They're looking for the drugs your parents were transporting."

"Shut up!" yelled the older guy.

"What?" hissed Jo. "What are you talking about?"

"I'll explain later."

The older guy, clearly the leader of their team, walked over to within an inch of Eli's face and said, "I don't want to have to tell you again. Shut....the fuck....up." He walked back to the other guy and then said to the men, "Ok, round everything up. Get rid of the raft. We'll cut the anchor lines when we leave."

The younger men pulled the raft into the trees and they began to load into the two red Donzi's.

"Move," said the leader, pushing Eli and Jo toward one of the boats. They got in and the younger guys handed their weapons to their friends before the pushed the boats off the beach.

The drivers started up the massive engines and with everyone on board, the two big boats motored slowly towards the *Bree-zee.* The guy sitting next to the driver reached out with a large knife and first cut the aft and then the bow anchor lines. The boats roared out towards the dark blue water of the Tongue of the Ocean, and Eli and Jo looked back at their last view of the *Bree-zee*, drifting helplessly towards the beach.

Chapter 15

"Where are they taking us?" shouted Jo. The roar of the engines and the wind rushing past them was so loud that Eli almost couldn't hear her.

"East," was all he could say.

He didn't know, but suspected they had a base somewhere in the northern Exumas. It couldn't be too far from Andros, since they would need to refuel. Besides, the nearest open water was Exuma Sound. That's where their "mother ship" was likely to transfer the drugs to the fast Donzi's, which could then reach various drop off and distribution points around the Out Islands.

"Why did you say that Mother and Father were transporting drugs?" Jo yelled.

"Because they were. How else do you think they ended up in this mess? Lloyd Taylor thought something fishy was going on with the finances. Where did you think the money came from?" Jo looked stupefied.

"They were bringing the stuff into Miami because the Customs agents knew your father or he'd bought them off."

Jo shook her head. "You're wrong, you must be wrong," she yelled. "Father would never do something like that."

Eli grabbed her hand and yelled into her ear. "He would if he was blackmailed into it."

She pulled back and stared at him with an angry but confused look. She turned her head away from Eli and looked out at the water as they flew by.

The boats were moving very fast, fast enough to go airborne when the crested the large swells of the deep water channel. Eli guessed more than fifty miles per hour, which meant that they were indeed making a run for the Exumas. *There's no way they're using Norman's Cay*, he thought. *But what if they are? What if they've set up shop again on Norman's Cay?*

It was a crazy thought, but it made sense. A first class landing strip, easy access to open water, years of inactivity. Maybe it was active again, just like Perry suspected. If they were headed there, they were in for a two hour ride. Eli sat back and stretched his legs. The guy in the seat next to him poked his gun into Eli's ribs and shook his head, so he sat up straight with his legs tucked in.

The bouncing of the boat and roar of the engines was numbing after an hour, and Jo fell asleep with her head bobbing against Eli's shoulder. She stirred when the boat impacted hard after the large jumps across the swells, but otherwise slept. After a little more than an hour, Eli could see the light green water of the shallow bank under them, and knew they would soon be at their destination. They continued at full speed for another thirty minutes and then he could see the islands just ahead. The lead boat headed for the channel between the Saddleback Cays and Norman's Cay, and their boat followed from a safe distance.

They slowed and Jo woke up abruptly, looking around and then at Eli. "Where are we?" she said, not having to shout.

"We're almost in," said Eli. "I think we're headed for Norman's Cay."

"Shut up!" yelled the guy in front. Eli's other seat companion again jabbed him in the ribs with the barrel of his MAC-10 for emphasis.

The boats motored slowly through the channel and weaved their way inside the barrier reef. They accelerated again for a few seconds before slowing suddenly. The first boat headed in towards shore and Eli could see a house set back slightly from the beach. It was beaten up pretty badly, missing wall boards and parts of the roof, but he recognized it right away. It was definitely Carlos Lehder's "Volcano House," so named for its massive cone-shaped fireplace built from the local limestone.

The Cubans beached the Donzi's and ushered Eli and Jo out and up to the house. They did not go in but instead walked around the house to the driveway, where a Ford Bronco with tinted windows sat with the motor running. A well dressed guy in his early thirties got out of the back and approached the older guy from Eli's boat. They walked a short distance from the rest of the group and the older guy explained in an animated way how they'd caught the two "tourists" and why they'd brought them in. The well dressed guy patted the older man on the shoulder and returned to the Bronco.

"Hey, guys. Let's go," said the older man to his younger colleagues, and they headed back down to the boats, leaving Eli and Jo alone with the younger guy and his body guard/driver.

"Please tell me who you are right now," said the guy in perfect English.

"Like I told your men, we were looking for the same thing you were," said Eli, staring into the guy's dark brown eyes.

"Yes, and just what was it that we were looking for?" The breeze blew the guy's thin black hair all over his eyes. He brushed it aside and looked at his gold Rolex.

"You were looking for the cocaine that the American couple was supposed to deliver for you. We came to collect it if we could find it and follow through with the deal." Eli prayed that the story was close enough to the truth to keep the guy interested.

"That's a very interesting story, Mister - I didn't catch your name."

"I'm Eli, this is Jo."

The guy smiled and extended his hand. "Well, Eli and Jo, my name is Manuel, and I don't have time to stay and talk. So I guess you're just going to have to take a little trip with me so we have the time to get to know each other better. Get in the vehicle, please."

The three squeezed into the back seat of the Bronco and they drove through the tree-covered driveway to the chain that blocked the entrance. A young guy let them pass and then they were off, driving quickly across the island and then south towards the landing strip.

"I'm surprised you're still using Lehder's house," said Eli calmly.

Manuel glanced at him and smiled. "So you know your way around, Mr. Eli? Well maybe you know too much. Maybe you are DEA, and you and your pretty assistant here are really just spying on our operation. Maybe I should just kill you here and not bother with you."

"I am NOT his assistant," exclaimed Jo. "I'm his employer. *He* works for *me*."

Damn, Eli thought. *Now she's done it.*

"Really. How very interesting. So tell me again, what is your name?" Manuel looked at Jo and smiled.

Realizing she'd said too much, Jo tried to back pedal out of the hole she'd dug, but to no avail.

"That's not important," she continued in an unconvincing tone. "What's important is, why are you holding us against our will? And your people back there, they damaged my boat."

Manuel laughed and shook his head. "Ok, let's leave this for the flight."

The Ford roared down the asphalt runway towards a waiting Learjet 31. "We are here. Please get on the plane and find a comfortable seat."

He let Jo and Eli exit and followed them to the open door. He waved at his driver, who waved back and turned the Bronco around. The driver parked next to the airport waiting area and the stewardess closed the door.

Eli was impressed. The plane was outfitted as an executive jet, with large chairs, a meeting table, and a sofa, complete with seat belts. He and Jo sat together on the sofa and put on their seat belts; Manuel sat in the large lounge chair opposite them. A stewardess greeted Manuel in Spanish and then asked Jo and Eli if they wanted a drink.

"Water would be nice," said Jo, and Eli requested the same. The stewardess went to the refreshment stack and returned with a rum and soda for Manuel and two bottles of water for his "guests." She announced, "Lady and gentlemans, please make sure your seat belt is close for the flight. We will be leave in just a few minutes." She then went forward to speak with the pilots.

"A toast to your health, Mister Eli and Miss Jo," said Manuel, raising his glass.

"Thank you," Jo replied. "And to yours."

Eli was not at all relaxed, as he knew that their struggles had only just begun. He smiled formally but did not drink. The pilot signaled their readiness for takeoff and closed the cockpit door. The jet's engines roared and they shot off down the runway, accelerating at high speed until they lifted off, not far from the water line. The plane banked right and flew low for a few minutes before they started to gain altitude. A quick look out the window confirmed that they were over Exuma Sound and headed southeast towards the Caribbean.

"So, my friends. Let's continue where we left off. And now we need to be open and honest about everything, yes?" Manuel looked at Jo.

Eli tried to size up Manuel but couldn't precisely place his accent. He'd probably learned English in the US, most likely California or Florida. He definitely wasn't a Cuban; more likely, he was Colombian, and he had a taste for good clothes. While his outerwear was not designer quality, it was likely still quite pricey - a pair of tailored cotton trousers and a white photographer-style shirt, the kind with numerous pockets and fasteners. His loafers were clean but not new, the Rolex and the chain around his neck were real gold, and his sizable ring appeared to hold a real diamond. *He likes shiny, flashy things*, he thought. *Unless he's gay he's going to like Jo.*

Jo looked at Eli, who nodded and said, "Why not?"

"Like I said, my name is Jo, really Josephine. Josephine McHenry. My father is.... was the CEO of McHenry-Taylor, the large fashion house. If you're kidnapping me then I suppose the Board will pay you a ransom, but I can't guarantee it." She sat back and sipped her water, looking at the young Colombian.

"Very interesting," he said. "So you are part of the family that Paco told me about." He considered his words for a moment and then said, "No, this is not a kidnapping. I didn't think that a ransom would be possible until you told me this, but now it may not be a bad idea. Maybe I can get one million dollars for you?"

"I should think so!" said Jo indignantly. Eli just rolled his eyes.

"And you, Mr. Eli. What is your name?"

"My name is Eli Rose. I run a private security business in Miami, and Jo here hired me to find her parents." He decided that the truth would be good support for the lies he would tell him next.

"Once Jo and I found out what was going on we headed over to look for the shipment. We know the deal her father made with Paco, so the idea was to do the same thing. We were going to drop it at the Hurricane Hole on Key Biscayne and tell Paco where to find it."

"Ah, I see. So you were going to honor the deal with Paco. And what happened?" Manuel leaned forward, focusing his attention on Eli.

"What happened was that somebody beat us to it. All we were able to find was the wreckage of the McHenrys boat. The coke was long gone. Then your guys showed up and started shooting, and the next thing we know, here we are."

"Here we are," repeated Manuel. He had an irritating habit of repeating the last thing said to him, and that was already getting on Eli's nerves.

"Ok, so maybe now it's my turn? My name is Manuel Durán. I am Colombian, but I was raised in California, as you surely have guessed, Mr. Rose." He smiled at Eli but the expression was not reciprocated.

"I attended university in Miami and received a degree in international business. Since my family is from Boyacá, I went home to work in the family business, which is ranching, but a better offer came to me while I was there."

"So now you work for Pablo Escobar," Eli said.

Manuel smiled and toasted Eli. "You are a very smart guy, Mr. Rose. Maybe you are too smart. Yes, now I have the responsibility to manage shipping for Medellín. As you observed, we use Carlos' old house from time to time just for meetings. We block the entrance and scare away the tourists when we need it. They have great stories and we don't stay, so there is nothing for the authorities to find there. I don't visit very often, but sometimes, like now, I have to come and check on things for myself."

"Do you have a bathroom on this plane?" interrupted Jo.

Manuel waved to the stewardess and said, "Please escort the lady to the lavatory and provide some privacy for her."

"Thanks," said Jo with a quizzical look. She got up and the stewardess walked with her to the lavatory. Since it was not enclosed it had been equipped with a curtain on a rod to pull around the toilet. Jo looked at the contraption skeptically while the stewardess demonstrated how to use it, then closed the curtain.

"Now that she's away," said Eli, "let's get down to it. We know the deal, so we're here to continue what was negotiated before, except I want a bigger cut of the fluff."

"Mr. Rose, why should I do something like that? What do you bring to the table that I don't already have without you?"

Eli leaned forward to make his point and replied, "Well, for starters, I'm bringing more to the table than just a boat. I used to be US Coast Guard, and I know their operating protocols and tactics. I know Miami as well as anyone and can find better ports of entry than the ones the McHenrys were using, plus I have friends in the RBDF that will turn the other way for a small fee. Will that work for you?" He had to use everything at his disposal in order to convince the guy they had some value. That was the surest way to stay alive.

Manuel smiled and uncrossed his thin arms. He looked almost too thin to Eli, like he was ill. But his strongly symmetrical face lent him the good looks and authoritative presence that he used to his advantage.

"Ok, Mr. Rose, let's say that maybe your proposal is of interest to me. We will of course have to work out the details, but maybe an arrangement like this will work."

Jo returned at that moment with a look of embarrassment and Manuel smiled. "So, you are refreshed now and ready for a long trip?" he asked.

"Yes. I'm sorry if anything disturbed you."

"No worries," said Eli. "We were talking and didn't notice anything."

Jo smiled and looked relieved. "So, Manuel......oh, I'm sorry. May I call you Manuel?"

"But of course."

"Thank you. Manuel, you said we have a long trip? Where are we going?" She glanced at Eli, who shook his head.

"We can discuss that later. Right now I need to tell you some things that may be of interest. I am telling you this because I am a sympathetic man, Ms. McHenry, and I don't think it is right for you to suffer, not knowing the fate of your parents. You see, the reason I came to the Bahamas is because of your parents."

"I don't understand," said Jo. "Please, can you explain what you're talking about?"

"Certainly." Manuel sat back, looking serious. "When your parents failed to show up at the scheduled drop off site, we sent some of our boats to look for them back where we made the exchange."

"You mean at the Joulters Cays." Jo was beginning

to piece things together as well.

"Exactly," he replied. "We were missing not only your parents, but the original boats and crews that we sent to meet them. The guys that found you, they also found our original team dead on Andros Island, and our boats were gone. Naturally, when they heard you were in Andros Town asking questions they waited to see where you would go. Since you went to the same place, they thought that maybe you were looking for the drugs. That's when they found you."

"But you said you had some more news about my parents?" Jo implored.

Manuel looked at her somberly and said, "We believe your parents are deceased, Miss McHenry. Our men found much debris from their boat, and we think they were ambushed and killed for the drugs."

Jo looked shocked but did not react the way she had on the island. "How can you be so sure about this?" she said.

"This is what has been happening," Manuel replied. "We have been using a distribution point in another country for the last few years. It has been very successful for us, but a couple of months ago the government of that country started to make things very difficult. We had to move the distribution point back to the Bahamas, to the Joulters area that you visited. We have been using this area for several years off and on, but recently we began to lose some shipments and other resources to pirates, and that is what we believe happened to your parents."

Jo sighed and looked at the floor. "That sounds plausible. I still won't be sure until I can prove it, but it's a reasonable scenario. Thank you for telling me that."

"It is the least I can do," said Manuel. "Now I suggest we relax for a time and enjoy the flight. We will be in Port of Spain, Trinidad in two hours, and we can decide at that time if we have business to do or not."

Eli knew that their Colombian host had not told Jo everything. He suspected much more and had pieced together the parts that Manuel had left out, especially the part about a future business arrangement. Eli knew that the Colombian had not told that story to Jo with the expectation that she and Eli would be set free. He had to convince Manuel that they were valuable assets or suffer the consequences, and he knew very well what that meant.

"All passengers will kindly fasten their seatbelts and prepare for landing."

The stewardess smiled as she walked back to check on the three passengers. The little jet bumped in the afternoon turbulence as the pilots began their descent to Piarco International Airport. Afternoon thunderstorms had begun to fire up along the Manzanilla coast and were rolling towards the west, and the pilots quickly maneuvered around a large one over Port of Spain and a second one that was rolling in from San Fernando.

Eli could see the verdant green mountains of the Northern Range as they glided in and then touched down on the rough asphalt of the runway. The little jet decelerated very quickly and turned onto the taxiway bound for the private plane hangars. Eli had arrived there once on a US government flight, but this was decidedly different.

The plane rolled to a stop and Manuel smiled. "So, we are here. Please follow me. I have a car waiting. He thanked the stewardess and walked down the small stairway to the tarmac, followed by Jo and Eli.

The afternoon air was as thick as soup and felt almost like a wet blanket had been thrown over them. Jo stood for a second to gather herself and said, "Is this Trinidad? I've never been here before. The mountains are beautiful." She seemed more relaxed and was in a much better mood than before.

"Yes, my dear Miss McHenry. Welcome to Trinidad, my home away from home. I hope you will enjoy your stay here." Manuel took Jo by the hand and led her to the middle one of three waiting Land Rovers.

"Don't we have to clear customs and immigration first?" she asked.

Manuel smiled. "That has all be taken care of. Please," he said, motioning for her to get in.

Eli followed, surveying the scene and recalling the images from his first trip there. The old terminal building was in a sad state and surely needed a rebuild, but the place was the same, small for its relative importance in the Caribbean and just as neglected. A small tow tractor was being connected to the Learjet's front wheels in preparation for transport to its home in a nearby hangar, so Eli followed Jo to the Rover and got into the back seat beside her.

Manuel spoke to one of his guards at another vehicle and the guy immediately got into a small Toyota Tercel and drove off. The other two Rovers were parked on either side and with a quick wave from the driver, one led the way and one followed Manuel, Eli, and Jo.

"Please accept my apologies, but I need to get back to my complex on the east side. Perhaps we can enjoy dinner in Port of Spain some other time."

Manuel seemed sincere but Eli knew the truth. If their story didn't check out they'd be dead by tomorrow evening. Not much point making dinner reservations for three if only one shows up.

"As you can see, we have a fair amount of security here. There is a lot of random crime on the highways these days, including kidnappings for ransom. Even I need to be concerned about such things." Manuel leaned over to Jo to explain himself better.

"The gangs that are involved in these activities here don't necessarily know who I am, and by the time they found out I could be in serious trouble. So we don't take any chances."

"It's that violent here?" she asked.

"Kidnapping is a growth industry in Trinidad. Mostly the gangs prey on local Indian businessmen and their families, since they own most of the businesses and have most of the money. But every so often a tourist or European national is in the wrong place at the wrong time and then there's trouble."

Jo shuddered and Manuel said, "Is the air conditioning up too high for you? I will have the driver turn it down."

"Thanks, that would be nice," she said with a faint smile.

"We will be going east to Sangre Grande, then south along the Cunapo Southern Road to my little paradise in the forest," added Manuel. "I will point out things of interest along the way, if you like."

She smiled weakly again, so Manuel continued to play tour guide while Jo feigned interest. Eli thought she might have finally understood the seriousness of their predicament, and that was what had darkened her mood.

§

The caravan drove north to the Eastern Main Road and then east at a high rate of speed, reaching Sangre Grande in about an hour. Slowed by traffic, they continued to the Cunapo Southern Road and then went south towards Manzanilla. Eli recognized the route as one he'd taken in the early 1970's when he was still working for The Agency. They had sent him to Trinidad to work with the local police to help root out the remaining Black Power revolutionaries and communist sympathizers that had gone into hiding after the 1970 revolt. He'd had the occasion to visit the east coast on some of his riskier field investigations, and had made some good contacts inside the American oil company, Amoco while there. He hoped that they might still be around, as he thought he'd need them very soon.

Traffic on the road south was bad for a Sunday, but that was mostly due to a couple of large trucks that could not pass very quickly along the winding, hilly road. Most of the heavy truck traffic was headed to Galeota Point, where Amoco had its main facilities. More than an hour after leaving Sangre Grande they had finally reached Mount Harris, the tallest point in the Central Range, according to Manuel, and a good point of reference for Eli. The lead Rover suddenly slowed and pulled off the road to the right, down a gravel-packed driveway. The other two vehicles pulled in as well and a passenger from the lead vehicle got out to open a large locked gate.

"We are here," announced Manuel. "Just a little bit farther and we will be at the house." The gate was unlocked and the first Rover drove through and pulled off the road to let the others pass. When all had entered, the guy closed the gate and the other vehicle followed.

They weaved slowly along the gravel road under the trees, which blocked out the remaining sunlight and cast a pall over the vehicles. They could see nothing except dense jungle on either side of the road and they continued on for another fifteen minutes until they reached a second gate. This one was opened from the inside, and upon entering they were surprised to see a large complex of low buildings. One was definitely a house, large but not ostentatious, while the others looked like staff lodging and warehouses. There was a large garage for the vehicles and electrical generation and water/sewer plants to provide independent sources of power and water. Eli remembered that he had not seen any power lines as they turned off the main road, nor water pipes for that matter.

The Rovers pulled up in front of the house and two guards opened the doors. Eli and Jo followed Manuel inside and they were surprised at how warm and brightly lit the space was, considering how dark and foreboding the jungle felt.

"Welcome to my home away from home," he said. "As you can see, we have tried to make it a comfortable place, so I hope you will relax and enjoy your stay with me. We will try and make it as brief as possible, since I know you wish to get home, Miss McHenry."

"That's very kind of you," said Jo timidly.

"I have asked Julio to make up a room for you. We have also managed to find you some clean clothes - not of great style, of course, but serviceable I hope. You can go and clean up and we will have a dinner at seven, if you are Ok with that?"

"That's great," said Jo. Julio led her down the right hallway and Manuel then turned his attention to Eli.

"Of course we've tried to do the same for you, Mr. Rose. But I would like to discuss a few more things with you before you go."

"Sure, Manuel. At your service."

Manuel led the way to the bar and offered Eli a stool. "What can I get for you?"

"An ice-cold Carib would be perfect about now," said Eli. The Trinidadian ale was surprisingly refreshing when served cold on a hot and humid day, and Eli had consumed his fair share of them on his last visit.

"Good choice. I think I'll have one as well." Manuel opened the large refrigerator and pulled out two bottles, then grabbed two frosted mugs from the freezer. "So,

Mr. Rose, tell me a little more about your work for the US Coast Guard. It sounds very fascinating." Manuel sat down and had a sip from his mug.

"There's not much to tell, really. I was a Lieutenant Commander in the 1970's and was put in charge of the drug interdiction program in Panama and Costa Rica. I helped develop some of the methods and protocols they use for inspections of cargoes, especially for ships at sea. From what I understand they have been using our recommendations very effectively."

"That's an understatement," said Manuel. "I would say that the Coast Guard has been very effective at finding what we try to conceal. Perhaps with your help we can change that."

"Perhaps."

"You know, of course, that I am checking on your story and tomorrow I will have some answers. Is there anything else you wish to tell me, just to keep the record straight?"

Eli contemplated how much to reveal. That he was working for Jo to help find her parents was already on the table and seemed to be accepted at face value. That he had friends connected with his Coast Guard service was Ok, especially since he knew he could count on them to play along with whatever came up. That he and Vicente were burrowing into the Medellín Cartel's distribution network in Miami was better kept a secret. Similarly, that he was a CIA contractor for fifteen years was also something that no one else should know about.

"Well, you'll probably find out that I've been in trouble in a few places, mostly doing the same type of job I'm doing now," he volunteered. "Otherwise, no.

There's nothing else."

Manuel put his beer down and stared at Eli silently for a few seconds. "Mr. Rose, let me tell you what I think. I think maybe you are a DEA agent with a really good cover story. I think you are a bullshit artist who thinks he can fool me by dropping a few names and fast facts. That's what I think." The Colombian was no longer smiling.

"*Señor* Durán, if you didn't think I had something of value you would have tossed me off the plane when we were half way across the Caribbean." Eli used all his resolve to act the part of wrongly accused criminal, trying at once not to offend him but also not to back down or show any weakness.

"Now let's cut to the chase so we can both get on with things. When your people in Port of Spain call you tomorrow they will confirm what I told you. Then it will be time to talk money and scheduling, and we'll have to move quickly to be able to keep our routes open. You know, the Cali Cartel has tipped off the Shower Posse about the routes and methods you're using right now."

The Colombian sat back on his bar stool, eyebrows raised with surprise. "Do go on, Mr. Rose. This is fascinating."

"Ok, I'll break it down slowly for you," Eli began. "Regardless of which mules you're using to move the loads from the Bahamas to Miami, Cali has a mole in your Miami network. I don't know who it is right now, but I can find out. They are tipping off the Cali boys, and the Cali boys stay clean by tipping off the Jamaicans. The Jamaicans hijack your mules and your crews when they catch them, and send the cargoes to their own distributors in New York and New Jersey. In this way, Cali get's what they want, which is to inflict damage to your organization, and the Jamaicans get free blow for the northeast market. You're the only loser in this game."

Manuel had a dour look on his face, almost a pained expression. "Suppose you are right about this. How do you suggest we counter the threat and still maintain our supplies to the US market?"

"You work with me. I can get you past the Coast Guard because I know how they work and what they look for. The Jamaicans don't know my routes and they won't know because all you're going to tell your Miami distributor is where the stuff is coming into South Florida. I'll use my connections, along with some of your cash to get us an escort from the RBDF while we're in Bahamian waters, and poof, your stuff has a clear transit into the area. But you have to turn the scheduling over to me, or I can't guarantee anything."

The Colombian reflected on what Eli said and the patted him on the shoulder. "I hope your story check's out, my friend. It sounds pretty good from here, and it may be worth letting you handle a shipment, just to see if it works." He smiled and squeezed Eli's arm.

"You know who you remind me of? Max Mermelstein. He was also a very confident guy, and for awhile he was very, very good and very useful to us. But in the end he turned out to be an informant, a traitor, and he hurt us very badly." Manuel sighed and added, "But you know, there are always ways to work around such difficulties, and that's how I see this one right now. We survived the loss of Max and Carlos and continued to grow. We will survive this as well."

He paused and stared straight into Eli's eyes, wishing to directly convey his threat without using the words to do so."Right now, the question in my mind is, which Max will you turn out to be? The useful one, or the traitor? We will see in the morning, after I've talked with Port of Spain. For now, why don't you go and get cleaned up for dinner? I think you and Miss McHenry have had a very eventful day."

"Sounds like a plan," said Eli calmly. Julio had returned and Eli followed him down the left hallway to a small guest room. It was plainly furnished but more than adequate, with a double bed, towels, and some clean clothes that looked like they might fit him.

"Do you need something Mister?" said Julio.

"No, thanks. This is great." Julio bowed slightly and closed the door as he left.

Eli took a deep breath and exhaled slowly. His demeanor hid the tension and stress he felt, knowing that his and Jo's lives depended on a background check and Manuel's desire to try something new. Regardless of the result of the call tomorrow, Eli had to find a way to get a signal to one of his contacts in Trinidad, or get a call out to Vicente. He was about to be put to the test to see how good a narco-trafficker he could be, and for now it looked like it was a test he'd have to pass.

Chapter 16

The place was a short walk from his apartment, less than two blocks. On Sundays his group of friends set up some tables in the shade next to the building and played dominoes until noon. Vicente found this very relaxing because the locale was so reminiscent of home - a heady aroma of strong *café cubano* mixed with *pasteles* and cigar smoke; the clatter of the dominoes being smacked against the table; the constant talk of politics and neighborhood gossip. Those mornings helped him reconnect with his roots and revitalize his soul.

It wasn't that he didn't like Miami. On the contrary, he *loved* Miami. But it wasn't Havana, and no matter how hard he tried, he could never quite feel at home away from his island birthplace. But he found Sundays at El Rey de Cuba cafeteria to be an acceptable substitute. Vicente was especially enjoying himself that morning, chatting with his old friends and telling lies. He was a respected member of the group; his reputation was widely known amongst his peers. Being a 2506 Brigade veteran *and* a member of Morgenthal's inner circle in Havana brought him instant credibility in the community, and on the occasions he felt like talking politics, everyone listened and nodded their heads in agreement.

It was just such a day for Vicente, a typical Sunday but one during which the conversation had turned to politics on the island.

"My cousin called me last night, you know, the one that works for the Ministry of Justice, and you know what he told me?" The old man paused and sat back in his chair, waiting for everyone at the table to take the appropriate notice.

After several seconds Manolo said, "Ok, Hector. What did your cousin tell you?"

Hector gathered himself and leaned in to speak in a low voice.

"My cousin told me that Admiral Martínez was arrested and will be put on trial for drug smuggling." He smiled with satisfaction, having revealed news he thought no one else knew.

"Bah, that's old news," said Manolo. "Everyone knows that he will end up the same as Ochoa."

Vicente's interest was piqued and he weighed into the conversation. "So, Manolo, you think he will be executed like Ochoa? Why do you think this?"

Now it was Manolo's turn to lean in and whisper. "Because the brother of my wife, who is in the Ministry of Foreign Affairs says that a successor has already been chosen. He is one of Raul's new boys, a very loyal guy, and someone Raul can trust. Besides, Fidel wants to get rid of the last of the old revolutionaries, especially the popular ones. That way there are no challengers in the future."

"That seems like a very good reason," said Vicente. "Has your brother-in-law heard any other stories about drug smuggling into Cuba?"

Manolo eased back and ran his good hand through his thin black hair. He re-lit his short, fat Fuente Hemingway cigar and sucked up a large cloud of tobacco smoke. He loved the acrid things but only smoked one per week, and only on Sundays because they were so expensive.

Vicente knew that when Manolo did this, he was about to reveal some deep, dark secret that most people didn't know. He also knew that this was Manolo's way of taking back the stage from Hector, his chief rival for bragging rights in their small group, but also his best friend.

"Of course, there are only rumors of these things, but my "sources" tell me that the Colombian cartels have infiltrated into the government by bribery, and they are able to move drugs through the ports at will. They bribe customs inspectors, security people, administrators, even the big commanders so that no one asks any questions. And everything was going fine until one of Martínez' men who was also taking bribes turned him in."

"And why would the guy do that?" said Hector indignantly.

"For immunity from prosecution," added Vicente. "But that's a waste of time because they will just kill him anyway. He will have an unfortunate "accident" in a few months."

The men all laughed and cigars were drawn like swords and smoked vigorously.

"So, Manolo, this is still going on, this smuggling?" asked Vicente cautiously.

Manolo puffed on the cigar. "No, I think now that things are quiet. There were too many people involved, and sometimes when it is like that there is a risk of someone, like Martínez' guy, tipping off the government. Raul has launched a big investigation of everyone connected with the ports and maritime security, and all the Colombian operations have been shut down."

Vicente smiled and folded his arms, having satisfied himself that his original information was correct. The Cuban ports were closed, at least temporarily, to the cartels, so they had to look for other means to trans-ship from Colombia. That was why Paco Gutiérrez had been so eager to accept Vicente's deal. *Paco must really be desperate,* he thought.

"Gentlemen, I am afraid it is time for me to leave you. Thanks for the great game and all the lies."

Vicente rose and hugged each man, patting them on the back. He walked back to the corner and the turned onto the sidewalk. *I bet the cartel has put a lot of pressure on Paco to keep the supplies flowing,* he thought. *Competition from Cali must be tough. Maybe that's why he blackmailed McHenry into doing his dirty work?*

He continued down the block and across the street. It was already a typical humid summer morning in Miami and there was no breeze, so Vicente's *guayabera* was beginning to stick to him like a second skin. As he crossed the street he saw a cable television repair truck parked in the parking lot of his apartment complex. *So*

Maria is finally having the cable installed, he thought. Still, it was a curious thing to see on a Sunday.

As he got to the metal stairway he noticed condensation dripping from his air conditioning unit. He instantly knew that was wrong. He'd turned the unit off when he left the apartment earlier that day, just like he did every time he left. *Someone is there*, he thought. Vicente went to the door and quietly tried the handle. It was locked, so he inserted his key in the lock and opened the door just a crack. There was no immediate reaction, so he prepared himself with a count to three, then put his left shoulder hard against the door and pushed in violently with all his strength. The door only opened half way before impacting something, *someone* on the other side. He heard a groan and rushed in to find a guy dressed as a cable repairman diving to the floor for a Smith and Wesson .38 Special.

Vicente kicked the guy in the shoulder and he let out a yell and fell over. He grabbed the gun and wheeled around in time to see another man, dressed in casual trousers and a light blue *guayabera* enter from the kitchen holding a Glock 22.

"Drop it," yelled the guy. Vicente lowered the revolver but did not drop it. The guy reached for his wallet and pulled it from his back pocket, flashing his identification.

"FBI. What the hell are you doing here?" said the angry agent.

"I live here," said Vicente, equally upset. "This is my place. What the hell *you* are doing here?"

The agent lowered his weapon and put his wallet back into his pocket. "We're finishing the install on your listening devices," he said, bending to help his fellow agent to his feet. "We didn't expect you for another hour."

Vicente handed the battered agent back his gun. "I sorry to hurt you friend here. He no give me much choice."

The guy rubbed his bruised shoulder and shook his head. "Nah, it's my fault for bein' so slow. I'm just finishin' up. Let me get my stuff." He went over to Vicente's telephone and started to put his equipment back into his toolbox.

"I'm Special Agent Rodríguez," said the other guy, shaking Vicente's hand. "How did you know we were here?"

"The air conditioner is on," said Vicente. "I always turn it off when I leave."

"Dammit, David. I told you we should have turned it off," said Rodríguez to his compatriot.

"Well it was too hot in here to work," retorted David, still rubbing his shoulder. "Why don't you cover the door next time like you're supposed to?"

"Gentlemen," interrupted Vicente, "have you finish you job? When does all this start?"

"We'll start monitoring your calls this afternoon, but in case we miss something you need to call us and let us know." Rodríguez handed Vicente his card. "You know the deal, so no games."

"Yes, I know the deal," said Vicente sarcastically. "Everyone has a deal."

"Just see that you honor ours," said Rodríguez. "You ready?"

"Everything checks out. Let's go," said David.

"We'll be seeing you around," said Rodríguez. He held the door for his injured colleague, gave Vicente a dirty look and left.

Vicente looked around his living room and did not notice anything out of place. *These guys are good*, he thought. The telephone seemed normal as well, though he found a bug when he unscrewed the receiver. He was just about to change his shirt and go get some lunch when the phone rang.
Can't those assholes wait even one hour? he said to himself. "Yes, this is Vicente. What do you want?"
The voice on the other end cursed him in Spanish, and Vicente knew he'd just jumped to the wrong conclusion.
"Listen, asshole. Paco is back and he wants to talk with you. Be at the corner of 3rd Avenue and 9th Street in thirty minutes. You know the car." The caller slammed the phone down, ending the call.
Vicente would have felt embarrassed if he'd been dealing with decent folk, but he still regretted not listening first before he reacted. *It must be the stress.*
His choices going forward were pretty clear: he had no desire to get cross-wise with Gutiérrez and his men, so as long as he kept his deal *in principle* with the FBI he didn't care if they liked him or they didn't like him. But he needed for Paco to like him, and he vowed to be more patient next time. He could not afford to have Paco angry with him.

Vicente decided to jump in the shower quickly and change into something more formal. Not a suit, but a better pair of trousers and shoes, and his best *guayabera.* He considered calling Special Agent Rodríguez to let him know what was happening. *Next time*, he thought. *We can start this afternoon.* Vicente put on a fair amount of Ralph Lauren cologne and locked the door, making sure it was securely locked this time. He walked over to the corner and stood there with his hands in his pockets, trying to look as casual as possible.

The black Mercedes roared up 9th Street from the direction of downtown Miami and the back door opened. "Get in," shouted the driver through his half opened window. Vicente complied and the car turned sharply down 3rd Avenue and headed towards 8th Street. Instead of turning to go east they continued on to 7th and turned left, heading west.

"We are no going to the house?" asked Vicente, suddenly concerned.

"The boss wants to meet you for lunch," was the reply from his back seat companion.

That meant only one thing to Vicente - they were going to the Versailles, and that was not good, not good at all. He started to worry. *They know me there. What if someone tips Paco?* He decided it wouldn't matter, since he'd already told him enough to blend in with his cover. But it would be a situation he couldn't control, where almost anything could happen, and that worried him.

The driver quickly maneuvered the big Mercedes down 7th Street, timing the traffic lights so that there were minimal stops. He took the turn onto 22nd Avenue and then the right onto 8th Street. From there it was a short ride to the restaurant and his rendezvous with Paco Gutiérrez. They arrived at the back parking lot exactly at one o'clock.

"Get out," said the guy next to him. Standing in full view of the street, the guy searched Vicente roughly, looking for a hidden microphone or a weapon. Finding nothing, the guy escorted him into the restaurant and pointed towards the back.

Vicente walked over and waited for Paco to notice him. "Your guys can be pretty rough when they want to be," he said. "They had me almost strip down in the parking lot before they would let me come in."

"And you think I like making them do this?" answered Paco. He waved for Vicente to sit with him. "I have to be cautious, old man. I can't let just anyone show up here and sit with me. So, did they look for a wire? Did the pat down get too personal for you?"

"Yes, and yes."

"Good, good. If you want to work for me you'll get used to it."

Vicente looked around and noticed that the restaurant seemed to be filled with Paco's "boys." Paco sat alone at a table in the back of the place, near the kitchen. *Most likely he can make a quick escape through the back*, Vicente thought.

"So, Paco, what's the occasion? All your guys are here. That can't be because of me?"

Paco laughed and slapped Vicente on the arm. "You are a funny old guy, you know that? No, this is a social thing. Every Sunday, I like to take the guys to lunch. It's my way of saying thanks. It's something extra for them and makes them feel good. You can call it "team building" if you want."

"Well thank you for thinking to include me, but I have still many things to do, so I will say thanks for the opportunity but.............."

"Sit down and shut up, old man!" shouted Paco. Several of his men and a couple of regular patrons raised their eyes to look but chose to ignore the outburst and continue with their lunches. Paco leaned in and said, "I tell you when you can leave. You do that again and I'll have one of the guys teach you some manners."

"Ok, Ok. No need to get upset," said Vicente, trying to defuse the situation. "I only meant that I still have some work to do to finish the preparations for the drop on Wednesday. It's for you, Paco. It's for you."

Paco sat back and smiled again. "Ok, old man, I get it. So let me tell you why I brought you here today."

The waitress walked over casually and interrupted with, "Ok, gentlemen. What will you have today?"

Paco gave the girl an angry look but said, "Give me the grilled snapper, and bring me some black beans and a *batido*."

She looked at Vicente. "And you?"

He didn't recognize her and that was a relief. "I would like the same," said Vicente. "Can I have fried yuca in place of the plantains? And water is fine."

The waitress wrote down the orders and said, "Thank you. I'll bring your drinks in a minute." She walked off towards the kitchen and Paco leaned in again to speak quietly.

"What I was saying was that we have a deal. The *Mexicanos* took only five minutes to decide. They want about four thousand five hundred kilos per week and they will pay one hundred thousand per kilo. We gave them a "new customer" discount for the first ten shipments, then they will pay one hundred fifty thousand per kilo for the next fifty shipments. We are sending one month's worth on this trip. Isn't that great?" He smiled and slapped the table.

Vicente nodded. "Congratulations. Yes, that is very good news. So everything will be ready for Wednesday?"

"Well, you see old man, we have a little problem. My people down south are saying now it will be Thursday night before we can get everything to Cuba. You will have to contact your people and have them ready one day later." Paco watched for Vicente's reaction to see how he handled the abrupt change in plans. Any sign of nervousness or uncertainty might throw his trustworthiness into question.

Vicente smiled at Paco and sighed. "Ok, Thursday night for the delivery. It will cost a little bit more because we will have to keep the workers overnight at the camp, but we can do it. Is there anything else?"

Paco eased back in his chair as their drinks arrived at the table. He sucked up the sweet milk shake through his straw and stirred it slowly.

"I'm glad to see you are a calm guy. That's good. You know the difference between someone who has balls and is successful and a guy who just has balls? The successful guy always keeps his head, no matter what is the situation. I like that about you, old man. You keep your head, no matter what."

Vicente studied his young partner but said nothing. He was supremely confident, sitting at a table in a neighborhood restaurant. But Vicente wondered how he would be in a fight, whether the guy would stand by his words or cry for his mommy when the shooting started. He hoped to never know the answer to that question.

There was one piece of unfinished business left for Vicente, and that was the issue of the McHenrys. He needed to risk asking Paco about it now, because it may be the last time he would have the opportunity.

"Paco, I need to ask you something, but don't worry if you can't or don't want to answer."

"Sure, old man. Ask me anything."

"I have a friend who is in the fashion industry, and he has some business with a guy that may be in some trouble. Do you know a guy called Donald McHenry?"

Paco scowled and threw his straw in his glass. The food arrived but Paco's expression didn't change, and he stared at the fish on his plate with disinterest.

"Another *batido* sir?" said the waitress.

"Sure, another *batido*."

The waitress smiled at Vicente and walked off to get Paco's drink. Vicente knew he'd poked the hornet's nest and he hoped it would be worth it.

"You ask me about this asshole?" began Paco. "Well, let me tell you something. This guy McHenry, he is a pussy, a worthless pussy. One simple job I give him and he never can get it right. Always complaining and giving me excuses. It was a mistake for me to bring him into this. Why are you asking me about this shit?"

"Like I said, I have a friend who is trying to do some business with his company."

"Ok. So tell your friend he is a stupid shit for wanting to do business with this guy."

Vicente continued to dig, a little deeper this time and slowly.

"So what happened between the two of you?"

Paco grinned and began to attack his fish like a *piraña*. "Here's how it started. One day about two years ago, one of my street guys, a good looking young *Cubano* who works the Bayfront Park area calls me to say he's met someone really important. This woman, the wife of a very big and famous businessman, just scored a few grams of coke from him near the marina. He saw her name when she dropped her wallet and her driver's license fell out. He just thought I should know. What a great opportunity! The wife of Donald McHenry, the famous fashion designer is scoring cocaine from one of my street dealers. I say to my guy, "Great. Keep track of how much she buys and how often you see her."

"So a few months go by and this bitch is scoring five, ten grams a week from him. He even starts to become friends with her and she starts to take him to lunch. So one day he tells me, "Paco, this lady is meeting me at noon and we will have lunch at the marina. We are getting to be really close, if you know what I mean, and I think maybe we will go back to my place after that."

"When I hear this, I say to myself, *This is a great chance to diversify the business.* You see, I'm always thinking like a businessman." Paco pointed to his head to signify his vast intellect. Vicente smiled and nodded, trying to pump up the kid's ego as much as possible.

"So I go to the marina and sit in a good place with my Nikon and my big telephoto lens. And I take photos, lots of photos. I take photos of the two of them laughing, and joking around, and then when she pays him and he gives her the package. All of it. Then I leave and go to his place and wait in the closet until they show up. And what the hell do you think happens?"

He paused, looking with anticipation at Vicente and hoping he will offer a guess. "I don't know. What happens?"

"You don't even want to take a guess? Not even one try?" Paco seemed disappointed.

"No, Paco. The story is too good. I cannot imagine."

"Fine," said the young guy, slightly disappointed. "So here's what happens. My young *chulo* starts to screw the shit out of this lady, and she is going at him like an animal, screaming like she's losing her mind. She's so into it that she never hears me taking the photos. Let me tell you, these photos were really something. I have not even seen this kind of shit in a porno movie!"

It was all very clear now to Vicente. It made him sick to put the whole picture together, but there was no other way it could have worked.

"I see. That must have been disgusting to watch. So you took the photos and the records of her buys to the husband to "persuade" him to do some work for you." He was happy to have a chance to use his new favorite word.

"That's a good word, "persuade." I like that. Yes, so I "persuaded" the old man to use his nice new sailboat to bring in some cargoes for me, since we needed to feed the demand here and our Cuba base was shut down. The guy did pretty good on the first trip more than a year ago, and he goes out a couple few times on his own and it's looking pretty good. But then all of a sudden he wants to start taking his wife on the trips, maybe to get her away from her *chulo* lover, and look what happens. He goes and get's them both killed! What a dumb ass! Plus, he gets some of my guys killed and we lose our boats. What a screw up. I guess there's not much I can do about it now. Then you come along with the solution to my problem. That's why I like you, old man."

Paco smiled and polished off the last of his fish and black beans and rice. Vicente had hardly eaten a bite, as he was totally immersed in the story the young criminal was telling.

"That is an amazing story," he said. "Too bad about the people, though."

"Screw them!" said Paco, belching for emphasis. "That asshole knew the risks. He wanted me to keep quiet, so I kept quiet. That was the deal, and I *never* break a deal. His part was to bring in the goods, that's all he had to do, and that worked until he screwed it up. Now it's over for him and his *puta* wife and it's no big loss to me. He was one of a dozen guys we have doing this shit, and so we lost one. Now we just move on to bigger things."

Vicente tried to comprehend what he'd just been told. The story made perfect sense and there was no reason for Paco to lie, since he didn't know about Vicente's connection to Jo McHenry. He couldn't wait to tell Eli what he'd learned.

"Ok, Paco. So let me go and get the word to the guys that we will be expecting the shipment on

Thursday night. Tell your captain that we will have one green light on the dock if everything is Ok and one red light if there is a problem. He can communicate with the dock on a frequency of 156.7 Megahertz. They will light the dock only when he has confirmed his arrival time. All of this has to be really fast so we don't attract the attention of the government. Is that Ok?"

'We'll hold up our end, old man. You just make sure your guys are ready."

Paco put down his drink and grabbed Vicente's hand. His thin, boney hand nearly disappeared into Vicente's but he squeezed down and added, "Remember, Vicente, no screw-up's. We get this right the first time or you end up feeding the fishes like the McHenrys."

Vicente smiled and nodded. "Not to worry my friend." He left his cold plate and went back to the waiting Mercedes for the ride back to his apartment.

Chapter 17

"I hope you are both refreshed and hungry," said Manuel with a smile. "The cook tells me we have king fish curry tonight."

"Sounds great," said Eli, sitting down next to Jo. *She doesn't look so good*, he thought. Jo wore the blue jeans and a simple blue shirt that she'd found in the room. Eli was happy to change out of his salt-crusted khaki trousers into jeans and a golf shirt, which was a little small in the shoulders but at least it was clean.

"Miss McHenry, tell me a little more about yourself." Manuel motioned for his housemaid to begin the service. "What are your interests? What are your plans for your father's company?"

"Those are distinctly different types of questions, Manuel. Well, let's see. My interests are pretty simple. I like water sports. I ski, swim, skin dive, that sort of thing. I enjoy good restaurants, I like to socialize with my friends." The maid distracted her by placing a bowl of green liquid on the table. "What's this?"

"Oh, that is a local specialty. It's a soup they call *callaloo*. It's really very good." Manuel ate some, almost as a gesture to signify that he was telling the truth.

"So that's really everything," said Jo.

"Very interesting," said Manuel without emotion. "And what types of drugs do you enjoy using?"

"Drugs?"

"Yes. What is your drug of choice these days?"

"I don't take drugs," Jo answered indignantly. "I would never do that. Not after.........."

"Not after what happened to your mother?" said Manuel slyly. He'd planned all along to maneuver her into this position, and now he moved in to press his advantage.

"Yes," said Jo, suddenly on the verge of tears. "That's right. Not after what she did. I would never do something like that."

Eli almost dropped his spoon into the soup. *So that's what started this mess?* he thought. *It was never Jo - it was her mother all along. That's why the old man was so easy to blackmail.* The puzzle was pretty much complete now, and he suddenly felt very sorry for his young boss.

"I think that is a wise decision. I do not understand the attraction so many Americans have for this crap," said Manuel. "You know, it's really crazy. We would have no business at all if your people didn't want so much of it. But cocaine is a lucrative business, better even than kidnapping and extortion, so we are happy to provide the product to whoever will pay us."

"But it's not all kisses and giggles for the cartels, either," added Eli.

Manuel looked away from Jo and stared at Eli for a

second.

"You are correct about that, *Señor* Rose. This is a very dangerous business because the amount of money we are talking about corrupts everyone it touches. We know this is a risk, but it's part of the business. So while we use this ugly thing to our advantage, we also fear it just the same."

"Manuel, why do you keep doing this? I mean, you are obviously very well educated and a smart guy. Is it just the money that keeps you involved, or is there more to it than that?" Eli was genuinely curious, but also hoped to find a personal connection he might be able to use to his advantage later.

"That is a very good question, and it's the first time someone ever had the nerve to ask me. But I am not offended, so don't worry." He paused and smiled at Eli, finishing his soup and waving for the main course to be brought to the table.

"To some extent it is the money, that's for sure. After this year I will have all I could ever hope to spend in ten lifetimes. But also, this becomes like family. It's really hard for me to explain, but we are a lot like the Sicilian Mafia in many ways. Once you become a member, it is like a family and you don't just quit your family. At least you don't do that and live very long." He smiled at the girl when she placed the fish in front of him and quickly changed the subject.

"So, Miss McHenry, what will be the future of the company, now that your father is no longer in charge? What do you think will happen to it?"

Jo looked down at the fish and then directly at Manuel, and replied with a steely-eyed stare, "I intend to run it the way I believe is best."

Manuel raised his eyebrows but continued to focus on the fish.

"That's an ambitious plan. My sources tell me that maybe the company will be a little short of funds in the next year. They also tell me that maybe your Board of Directors will move to sell the company if there is no one to present a good alternative to the financing problems. How do you think you will be able to keep your company?"

"I don't know right now," she said considering the question carefully. "I'll think of something."

"Can I offer a suggestion?" said Manuel, pausing to look at her. "We would be willing to invest in your company and we can offer you a very good deal."

"What sort of deal?" she asked.

"We could maybe contribute one hundred fifty million right now, and if things work out, maybe another one hundred fifty million by early next year."

Jo was stunned by the numbers. Eli wasn't at all surprised, and knew exactly what the drug dealer wanted.

"You would be willing to put up three hundred million? And what would you want in return? That's about fifty five percent of the value of the entire company, Manuel. You're asking me to turn over control to you?"

"Not exactly," he said. Manuel seemed distracted, almost disinterested as he used his knife to push leftover pieces of fish around his plate.

"What I would propose to you is that you let me fund your operations for a year. Obviously, you have to pay me back, so we have to work out a payment schedule. We can give you the same deal we offered to your father - you keep ten percent as a "fee" for administering our investment, and deposit the remaining two hundred seventy million at regular intervals in one of our Cayman accounts. I think that will be fair."

Eli shook his head and that attracted Manuel's attention. "So your employee here does not think this is such a good idea," said Manuel. "What do you think?"

Jo took a deep breath and Eli was sure he knew she'd say no. "Your offer is very interesting, Manuel. May I think about it until tomorrow?"

Eli was floored and couldn't help himself. "What? Jo, that's money laundering. He just wants to use McHenry-Taylor as a means to legitimize the cartel's earnings. You're not really going to do this, are you?"

She glared at him and put her fork down before she spoke.

"Eli, of course I know it's money laundering. I wasn't born yesterday. And you have no idea how hard it is trying to keep a company going. In my case, the company was built by my father from his own ideas and sweat and hard work. He did anything he could to keep from losing control of it, and I don't blame him one bit. If he'd let me step in when it was time he never would have been in the situation he was in. So what am I going to do? I don't know right now. I just need some time to think about it."

"Yes, of course Miss McHenry. That will be no trouble at all." Manuel smiled, satisfied he'd sprung the trap at the right time.

"Manuel, if you'll excuse me, it's been a long stressful day and I'm very tired. I think I will go and get some rest."

"Certainly," he replied. "Before you go, let me tell you that tomorrow at eight in the morning we will go up to my base on the north coast, so please be ready for breakfast at seven."

"Fine. Thank you for your hospitality, and good evening."

The two men stood while Jo left the table and Manuel approached Eli. "Let's go have a drink in the living room."

Eli followed him into the room where one of his men waited for orders. "Julio, get me a glass of the Macallan please. And for you *Señor* Rose?"

"Nothing thanks. I'd like to have a clear head for tomorrow."

"As you wish. There are some questions I would like to ask you about how your Coast Guard operates."

Eli knew he'd eventually have to discuss the subject, but he hoped he'd have more time to consider his story. Unfortunately, his time was up.

"Sure, Manuel. What can I tell you?"

Julio handed a glass to Manuel, who then said, "Julio, bring me the map, please. I want to have a better idea of what to expect when we are moving cargoes around in various areas, so I have several questions. For example, what are the most patrolled parts of the Caribbean? What routes should I take versus the ones I should stay away from? How does the Coast Guard work around the Gulf of Mexico? How frequent are the spotter flights and where do they concentrate their efforts? Those types of questions."

Eli had no intention of giving Manuel the type of operational details he wanted, but he had to give him enough information so that he wouldn't appear to be holding back.

"And what's my incentive for telling you anything? You won't really need me around if I just dump everything to you, now will you?

"I suppose you are correct," said Manuel. He put his feet up on the polished teak coffee table and relaxed into his overstuffed leather chair. "But I could take the information from you if I wanted to. You know this, so why don't we make this easy for both of us."

Eli considered grabbing a knife from the table and killing the smug Colombian while he could, but that was not a long-term solution to his problem.

"I will tell you a few things now but you have to work with me. Remember, I can get your shit through the Bahamas and South Florida every time."

"So you say," said Manuel. Julio returned with the map and Manuel thanked him. "Now you can prove it. Tell me where I should not go right now."

Eli felt like he had no choice but to give the guy something.

"Ok, this is what I'm comfortable telling you right now." He pointed at the map of the northern Caribbean.

"Whatever you do, stay away from the northern area, up here. The Coast Guard patrols this area with four WPB-110 Island Class cutters, two big WMEC-270's, and one WMEC-210. I know some of those guys - they're really good. They also use HU-25A Guardians to fly the area and they're out all the time, so going north is a bad idea. The southern route is much less risky."

Manuel, now keenly interested, stared at the map. "Why is the southern route less risky?" he repeated.

"Because the 110's are having multiple hull problems in heavy seas, including breaches. They don't want to risk them out in the central Caribbean, and their range is limited anyway. It would most likely be the 270's and the 210 that you'd find out there, and they're easy to keep tabs on."

"So how would you recommend we go?"

"My recommendation is that you slide whatever vessel you're using up the east coast of Yucatán and then head for the Windward Passage. But keep in mind that if there is a cutter in transit to Guantanamo Bay, you could get surprised. It's happened before, but I can find out from my contacts if there are any in the area, so I can pretty much guarantee we can avoid them. Once we get into the Bahamas we'll need to watch out for the RBDF, but like I said, I can find out about their patrols. They are pretty limited in what they can bring to the table anyway, from the perspective of equipment. After that we are in small boats, and all we have to do is watch out for 110's like the *Sitkinak* that are based in Key West or Miami Beach. They run eleven of those things in the coastal waters around South Florida, so using large ships is a real mistake."

"Yes, we already know this. The Cali boys lost a cargo a couple of years ago in the Windward Passage but that was because they didn't have someone like you around, who knew when the cutters would be on patrol. Nevertheless, we are trying one more time along the same route where you and the lovely Miss McHenry were picked up. We'll see soon if our misfortune was just bad luck or truly something more. In the meantime, we have another plan, which I may tell you about tomorrow, if your story holds up."

Eli relaxed. He realized he'd just demonstrated his value to his host. "Ok, sounds interesting. By the way, I heard about that seizure. It was a cabin cruiser with some poorly disguised compartments in it, right? They had the bad luck of running into the cutter *Tampa* while she was on a routine patrol. Amazing that no one ever looked for the cutter."

"Well we do not have the knowledge that you obviously posses. I am impressed, *Señor* Rose. Maybe I did not give you enough credit. We will soon see. Anyway, this has been a very interesting evening for me, but I am afraid I must get some rest. Tomorrow will be a very busy day for all of us."

"Yes, of course," said Eli. Julio led Eli back to his room and locked him in. He laid down on the hard bed and contemplated how he might get himself and Jo out of the horrible situation they were in, but fell asleep in a matter of seconds.

Chapter 18

The thunder was deafening. It reverberated through his head like the sound of a bass drum, but it seemed detached from the scene around him yet still strangely part of it. Eli suddenly realized it was a dream, and the sound of thunder was actually Julio pounding on the door.

"Is seven, *Señor*," he said. "You must wake up."

"Ok, Ok, I hear you," answered Eli, groggy. He pulled on his jeans and shirt and opened the now unlocked door, stopping off in the bathroom before accompanying Julio to the dining room. Jo and Manuel were already eating when Eli arrived, so he smiled and sat down silently, listening to the dialogue.

"Ah, *Señor* Rose, so happy you could join us. I was beginning to worry about you."

Manuel continued to eat his *buljol*, a mix of saltfish, peppers, tomatoes, and eggs that he shoveled in at a rapid pace with the assistance of his *fry bake*, a type of fried cornbread. Jo picked at her plate, nibbling a few bits here and there but appeared disinterested.

"No need, Manuel. I wouldn't miss the party for

anything."

Manuel looked up from his plate and smiled.

"I thought as much. I will have a surprise for you today. Besides the beautiful scenery, I will have the chance to show off one of our newest toys. I think you will like it."

"I can hardly wait," Eli answered, munching on a *fry bake* and gulping down a cup of strong Trinidadian coffee. "Have you heard from your sources in Miami yet?"

"No, but it's still early over there. I don't expect to hear anything until we get to the Matelot base. You're not worried, are you?"

"Not at all," Eli lied. "I'd just like to get that part behind us so we can do what we came here to do."

"Fine," said Manuel, laying his fork beside his plate. "Then I suggest we get to it."

He stood up and waved for Julio to get his guards moving. "Shall we?" He motioned for Jo to follow Julio, so they all exited the house and went out to the waiting Land Rovers. The doors were already open with the motors running, and Jo and Manuel got into the back of the middle vehicle. Eli looked quizzically at Manuel for a second but realized he was not welcome, so he opted for a seat alongside the driver of the first Rover. The vehicle had been converted to a left-hand drive model, which was unusual for Trinidad, so Eli sat to his right.

He guessed that Manuel would use the travel time to Matelot to convince Jo to take his "funding" deal. Jo would be easier to convince away from Eli's influence, and there was no way of predicting what she'd do. He could see that he really didn't know her very well, and his understanding of her motivations was no clearer now then it had been when they first met.

The caravan motored back to Sangre Grande where they turned northeast onto to the Toco Main Road. Once out of town and away from the tangle of *maxi taxi's* and delivery trucks, they picked up speed and drove off towards the coast. There was nothing for Eli to do along the way but think about how he could get himself out of the trouble he was in. Unfortunately, he realized that escaping into the jungle of the Northern Range with or without Jo wouldn't necessarily guarantee him a successful outcome. The terrain was very rough and there were no settlements to speak of in the higher parts of the mountains. He'd be out of contact with the authorities for days, even if he did survive the trek. There had to be a better option. *Maybe I can get some ideas by discussing the route with Arthur?* he thought.

The driver of his vehicle was a Trinidadian, and Eli knew this only because one of the other drivers had referred to him "Cokee-eye" Arthur. That slang term was the unflattering way the locals referred to someone who was cock-eyed or cross-eyed, and in that regard, Arthur certainly fit the description. He was a big guy, with the long dreadlocks typical of a Rastafarian, and with a right eye that peered outward away from center. He sat silently as he drove, his huge hands lightly gripping the steering wheel and making it appear half the size it really was.

"Arthur, how far is Matelot from here?" said Eli abruptly.

Arthur sat silently but his right eye stared in Eli's direction.

"I've been up there, to the north coast before, but it's been a long time. Those places like Toco Bay are really nice compared to the touristy beaches out west."

Arthur was silent for a moment but then answered, "So yuh tink yuh know 'bout we country?"

"I was in Trinidad a long time ago, but I enjoyed my visit. So where are you from?"

"San Fernando. We family from de area pretty close by." The right eye stared at Eli but the left eye still focused straight ahead.

"Dis' place we go now, Matelot. Is uh great place for a lime uh fete at de beach. But we eh goin' tuh no fete der."

"What is there?" asked Eli.

"Hmm. Yuh really doh know?" A smile crossed Arthur's face, the first time Eli had seen anything but a scowl since they'd left.

"Yuh gon see we base der, all de operation what it be. We got a house in Matelot and nothing more. De main show be up de coast."

Eli had his wish, but now he needed to slide the conversation more towards what he hoped would give him something he could use for an escape.

"So it's an impressive operation that Manuel runs up there, eh? Don't the locals ever get curious about what's going on? How does he keep it all a secret."

Arthur laughed. It started as a slow, quiet rumble, then filled the front of the Rover like a bullhorn.

"We doh get no maco's der. A maco be a curious person. Most people, dey know tuh stay away."

"I see," Eli replied. "Makes sense. Hey, by the way, how do you get along with these guys?" He pointed to the two Colombian guards in the back seat, now asleep and snoring enthusiastically.

Arthur smiled again and said in a low voice, "We Trini's got uh sayin' - all skin teet eh laugh. It means, be careful uh de guy dat smile too much; maybe he stab yuh back. Deez guys be mooks. You doh trust 'em as far as yuh can tro' dem."

"So let me ask you something, just between us. If I needed to get back to Port of Spain in a hurry, what's the best way for me to do that?"

The big driver stared at Eli with both eyes for a moment and nodded his head. "Yuh not one uh dem, right? Who yuh be, man?"

"I'm just a guy trying to get home," said Eli. He sensed something about Arthur that was different from the others, something encouraging, maybe even sympathetic to his plight.

"Ah see," said Arthur quietly. "Maybe all yuh best be close by mih today." He nodded his head again and looked over at Eli with his good eye.

Eli understood. Whatever Arthur was talking about was probably not part of Manuel's plan, and that change was likely to be forceful enough to change the dynamic in the group. He decided to heed the big Trinidadian's advice, and he would make sure that Jo was within an arm's length as well.

The drive from Sangre Grande to the north coast is

about as draining and tedious as anyone could ever imagine. The road winds along the northeast coast in a long series of curves and small straight-aways, and the views of the open Atlantic and the sea cliffs can be majestic in places. But the vistas quickly begin to merge into the same view after the first hour, and one loses track of time on the two-lane, rutted asphalt.

Just after the village of Redhead the road begins to climb the eastern corner of the Northern Range, and the welcome change in topography rewards the diligent traveler with views of the heavily forested mountains and valleys to the west. It then branches west at the village of Toco where it becomes the Paria Main Road, and passes through a seemingly endless set of curves through dense forests that close in around the road like a shroud. From time to time there are breaks through the trees and a spectacular view of the coast can be had. But the road soon plunges again into the green cover of the forest, and is broken only by small towns like Sans Souci and Grande Riviere.

Arthur pulled over to let the other vehicles pass as the caravan entered Grande Riviere. The new lead vehicle pulled into a small rum shop and stopped, and the other Rovers followed suit. The drivers, guards, and passengers all jumped out to stretch and buy refreshments. The two Colombians in the back seat of Eli's vehicle woke with a start but quickly collected themselves, jumping out to converse with their mates. Eli saw Manuel point towards the outhouse behind the building and Jo headed for it with a keen sense of purpose. A couple of the other guards relieved themselves by the side of the building while Manuel walked past them and into the building with a disgusted look.

Eli bought himself a Coca Cola and a Peardrax, or Pear "D" for Arthur, who remained at his vehicle throughout the stop. The fizzy liquid was certainly cold but too sweet for Eli's tastes, but Arthur thanked him and guzzled it down in just a few deep gulps. Eli returned the bottles and leaned against the Rover, waiting for the procession to begin again.

"Arthur, I don't mean any offense by saying this, but you seem like too nice a guy to be part of this gig. What's your story?"

"Ha, ha, yuh uh funny guy, Eli. Ah guess is uh fair question tuh ask. Is uh job, man. An de big pappy, he pay good. In troot, mih uh God-fearing man an ah doh like de drugs. Dey bad fuh yuh. Maybe ah is leavin' real soon, go back tuh Central an work on de coco plantation. Is hard work but honest, is so?"

"Is dat, Arthur, is dat." Eli smiled.

Arthur grinned broadly, his good eye focused on Eli, and he extended his right hand through the window. "Yuh alright, Eli." They shook hands, though for Eli it was more like having his hand swallowed by a catcher's mitt. "Remember, stay close later."

Jo emerged from the outhouse and returned to the second Rover, where Manuel handed her a Coke. Everyone got back into the vehicles and they started off towards Matelot. The road wound again through the dense forest before it finally broke free and skirted the hills near the ocean. Eli could see small settlements and isolated beaches and coves around every turn, an attractive scene for a tourist looking to get away from the usual resort-island frenzy.

A quick curve to the left soon revealed the first homes and small businesses that made up the tiny village of Matelot. It certainly wasn't much to look at; a few newer structures but most were no more than weather beaten, poorly constructed shacks. The caravan turned off the main road and headed back into the foothills of the nearby mountains, following a dirt road a few hundred feet to a small complex of buildings. Eli noted a storage facility, a main house, and some smaller houses that he guessed were staff quarters, essentially a smaller version of what they visited to the south near Mt. Harris.

The Rovers pulled in next to a large house and Manuel and Jo got out. Eli accompanied them inside while the guards and drivers milled around outside. Their stay would obviously not be too long, since the drivers left the motors running in the vehicles.

"Please have a seat at the table, my friends," said Manuel with a wave of his hand. "I must make a couple of quick telephone calls, so I will be with you shortly. Please excuse me." He walked off towards a back room while Eli and Jo sat at the long teak table.

"I trust you enjoyed the ride, *Señor* Rose," Manuel called out.

"Yes, very entertaining," Eli replied.

"Good, good. Glad you enjoyed it." Manuel immediately changed to Spanish and spoke more quietly, so Eli turned his attention to Jo.

"I guess you had quite a cozy ride with our host," he said, trying to provoke her.

"And what's that supposed to mean?" Jo was angry and he could see she had likely been unhappy for awhile.

"Just that you and "*Don* Juan" seemed to be getting along pretty cozy from what I could tell. So did you accept his deal?"

"That's not your business," she answered, indignantly. "Manuel can be very persuasive, but nothing's been decided, if that's what you want to know."

"Ok, sorry to get you all riled up. Listen, while we have a second alone I need to tell you something. One of the drivers has been telling me to stick close to him if I want to get out of here. I don't exactly know what's up, but I'd like you to stick with me in case something happens."

"In case what happens?"

"I don't know, but it didn't sound like it was something Manuel was planning, that's for sure."

Eli heard the call end and put his finger to his lips to silence Jo. Manuel returned with a stack of maps under his arm and a big grin.

"So, Eli, you will be happy to know that your story has checked out with my people in Miami. Now I feel I can share some more details with you about our operations so that you can advise me if we are doing something that is too risky." He laid the maps on the table and started to spread then out so Jo and Eli could see.

"This is a map of the Orinoco River in Venezuela. Let me show you what we do right now, and tell me if you see any holes in the plan. We use barges on the

Orinoco to ship our cargoes from Colombia. We land them in Ciudad Guyana and store everything in the warehouses near the port facilities. When we have enough for a large shipment, usually two or three barges worth, we transfer everything to *pirogues* we buy here in Trinidad and take them up Caño Macareo to Punta Pescador. What do you think so far?"

Eli was impressed with the plan. No question that the Venezuelans would not work too diligently to search Colombian barges, especially if the customs agents were paid off, and taking fast, maneuverable Trinidadian boats through the Delta Amacuro to Columbus Channel was a masterstroke.

"Great plan," he said, genuinely. "So what do you do with the stuff when you get it here?"

Manuel smiled, satisfied with the positive feedback from Eli.

"Sometimes we land the cargoes at Manzanilla Point if the sub is not ready to go. If it is ready, we take everything here."

"What did you say?" said Eli. "Did you just say the word "sub?"

"I knew I would surprise you sooner or later," said the Colombian with a grin. "This was all my idea, but it was difficult at first to get Pablo to go along with it. It cost us a huge amount of money, but it has been paying off until just recently. Yes, my friend, we have purchased a submarine. But not one of these small things that cannot cruise long distances."

"Ok, Manuel, what do you have?"

He beamed and pointed to a map of the north coast area, close to where they were.

"It's quite a story," he exclaimed like an excited child. "You see, more than a year ago, my connections with the Russian Mafia mentioned that they could purchase a functioning nuclear submarine from the Russian navy, including the crew. Of course I didn't believe them at first, but they insisted they could deliver it, minus the weapons of course. It would need a refit and some replacements for some key crew that wouldn't agree to leave Russia, but those were minor points. We agreed to exchange cocaine for the sub so we were not out much cash in the deal. It was about one billion dollars worth of product, but it was a steal! Look, here is a photo. Isn't she beautiful?"

Manuel pulled a photo of the submarine from the stack of maps and put it on the table. Jo stared at it with her mouth wide open and Eli was equally stunned.

"It is an OSKAR-1 Class, the K-173 *Krasnoyarsk* so they tell me, but I am not sure of this. We had to refit the hull in several places and update the batteries, but it works very well. We keep it in West Africa when it needs maintenance and refueling, or the crew needs a break. The Russians had already removed the torpedo and missile rooms so we could expand the storage, and now we can take many tons of cargo on each trip north."

Eli was speechless. He remembered hearing from his Coast Guard buddies that the OSKAR-1 Class submarines were the third largest nuclear submarines ever built, trailing only the Russian Typhoon and US Ohio Class subs. To acquire one of them was almost unimaginable, but he'd also heard that several of the recently   decommissioned   versions   had   gone unaccounted for. He always wondered what had happened to them - now he knew, at least as far as this one was concerned.

"I can see you are impressed. That is one of the reasons I wanted to bring you here. We are in the final stages of loading our next cargo, so you can go with me and see how we do things."

Manuel was delighted with himself and the reaction of his guests. He collected the maps and shoved them into a folder. "We must go if we want to catch the sub before it leaves."

Eli and Jo got up and went out with Manuel to the waiting vehicles, which drove off towards the beach. A small dirt road led to a parking area where the large Rovers pulled over and stopped. Before Eli could exit the vehicle, Arthur said to him in plain English, "Remember what ah say when yuh come back. No second chances."

Eli nodded and got out of the Rover. He met Jo and Manuel at their vehicle and Manuel told his head guard to wait for him with all the men. They then walked a few feet to the path that led down to the beach and a waiting *pirogue*, which was pulled up on the sand. The captain of the sleek boat was at the controls and had the motors running, while his first mate secured a small ladder to the sand so the guests could board without getting soaked by the surf.

Clouds were building over the center of the island but the north coast was free of rain for the moment. The intense sun beat down and burned them quickly, so the three moved back under the Bimini-style cover next to the captain. The mate threw the ladder onto the boat and then pushed off while the captain revved the motors in reverse. The boat slipped easily off the beach and was cutting through the waves and out to sea in a few seconds. The mate opened a cooler and offered them a selection of cold drinks, everything from beer to juice. Jo and Eli each grabbed a water, taking advantage of the opportunity to have something available later if it was needed. Eli stole a second bottle, wary of Arthur's warning and not wanting to be caught without supplies again.

The boat turned around the point and headed southwest along the coast, staying just north of the large rocks that lay offshore. After a short but bumpy ride they arrived at a small cove with very steep cliffs on the west and south sides and a pair of small islands on the right. Tucked between the islands and the west shore of the cove was the sub, a dark grey cigar-like shape that held position while a *pirogue* offloaded the last of its cargo. Manuel waved at the captain of the sub, a young-looking blond-haired guy in a Russian naval uniform and he waved back with a smile.

"He's ready," said the Colombian, and the sub crew completed their loading operations and then disappeared into the tower as the *pirogue* backed away from the sub. The huge ship moved forward slowly and began to submerge close to Manuel's boat, but was under before it reached them. Eli could see it descend through the clear water until it had slipped past them into the deep water offshore.

The captain of Manuel's boat then turned around and headed back towards the beach where he'd picked up his guests. Eli and Jo sat together silently as the boat bounced through the swells. He was stunned, and he wondered how the US government would react when the intelligence services discovered that the Colombian cartels had just become a naval power.

Chapter 19

"Oh, dear God! Something happen to them, I know this." Vicente was distraught when Leslie Robertson told him his Andros patrol had found the *Bree-zee* beached on Joulters Cay.

"Vicente, I promise, we are doing everything in our power to find them. If they are still in the Bahamas, we will locate them. You need to trust me on this." Leslie sounded sincere but Vicente could tell he didn't have a clue where Jo and Eli were, or even if they were still alive.

"Ok, Leslie. I know you do what you can. I wait until you tell me something. When you will call again?"

"I will call Rita back this afternoon. Don't worry, we'll turn up something by then, I'm sure of it."

"Ok, Ok. Thank you very much. Goodbye." Vicente put down the receiver and stared at Rita, whose eyes already welled with tears. "He say that maybe they know more later in the day. He will call you late, so no go home early today."

Rita's makeup was streaked by her tears and all she could do was nod and reply softly, "Ok. I'll be here."

"I go to my office to make some calls," said Vicente, who walked off slowly with his shoulders bowed. He went in and closed the door and sat down as if the weight of the world was on his back. He put his feet up on his desk and stared out the window for a while, lost in thought. Without word from Eli it was hard to know what to do. Should he continue to string Paco along or just turn him in to the DEA and be done with the whole affair?

Vicente decided to call Special Agent Rodríguez and tell him the entire plan. He'd already got to the bottom of the McHenrys sordid affairs and likely knew what had become of them, so there was little else to achieve at this point. He dialed the number on the card the agent had given him and the agent said, "Yes. Are you ready to talk?"

"I have some things to tell you," said Vicente. "When can we meet?"

"One hour. Go to the torch and admire the plaques." The call ended and Vicente looked at the receiver as if it had broken. He put it back in its cradle and went back over to Rita's desk.

"I go to have an early lunch. I will be back here in two hours." Rita just nodded as he left the office.

Vicente went down to the garage to retrieve his car, all the while feeling as though he was being watched. He couldn't exactly tell from where, but someone was definitely observing his movements and it made him very nervous. He drove down Biscayne Boulevard and parked at one of the meters across the street from the Torch of Friendship. He tried to blend in with the rest of the tourists by waiting with the crowd for the cross walk light to signal he could cross to the bay side of Biscayne Boulevard. He walked across with a group of German tourists and pretended to look back at all the high-rise buildings as if he was seeing them for the first time. Then he casually approached the monument and began to inspect the plaques for each country, starting with Mexico. It always pained him that Cuba was not one of the countries represented on the wall, but it no surprise why it had been left off. *Maybe one day*, he thought.

One of the Germans asked him in poor English if he would take a picture of he and his wife in front of the Kennedy Memorial, so Vicente graciously complied. As he was handing back the camera he felt a tap on his right shoulder and turned to see Special Agent Rodríguez standing next to him, dressed very casually in a white *guayabera* and khaki trousers.

"Let's take a walk," said Rodríguez.

They began to stroll through Bayfront Park until they were off by themselves, walking along the bay at the southeast end.

"I did some homework on you," the young agent continued. "I know who you are, what you've done. You're a pretty impressive guy, a real Cuban patriot. Even my grandmother has heard of you."

"That is very flattering," answered Vicente.

"Seems like you're held in the same esteem as Jorge Mas Canosa and Manolo Reyes. Many people tell me you're a veritable God, you can part the seas like Moses with just a wave of your hand. But I'm thinking maybe not. I'm thinking maybe it's all an act and you're really just another low-life drug runner like the rest of Paco's guys."

Rodríguez was agitated and not at all happy about having to talk with someone he felt was just a parasite on society."Prove me wrong, Vicente. What have you got for me?"

In his younger days, Vicente would have reacted in a very bad way to having been called a low-life and a parasite on society. His activities with Morgenthal notwithstanding, he'd led the life of a patriot and had made sacrifices that his young minder could never imagine.

"I will tell some important things about you friend Paco Gutiérrez and the deal we have," he said. "But first, let me ask you - where you are born?"

Rodríguez rubbed his closely shaven head and said, "Ok, I'll play. I was born in Miami. Why do you care?"

Vicente smiled. "You no have been part of *La Lucha*, my friend. You know what you parents and grandparents tell you, but you come from this country and this society. You no understand me or my life so you no judge me."

The young agent stared at him silently for a moment. "Fair enough," he replied. "I'll try and keep an open mind, but don't waste my time here."

"Very good. So now I tell you something."

Vicente recounted the events of the past few days in great detail; what he and Eli were hired to do, how he'd gained access to Paco's inner circle by arranging the offloading in Pinar, where and how the shipment would arrive in Mexico. But he left out the part about the submarine. He'd save that for Morgan.

Rodríguez pulled a small note pad and pen from his shirt pocket and furiously scribbled notes while Vicente relayed his tale. After the older man finished, Rodríguez said, "Ok, Vicente, that's a very interesting story. I need to ask you some questions before we go. How are the drugs getting to Cuba?"

"By sea, but I no have information on the route." That was at least partly true.

"When do you meet up with Paco?"

"We meet on Thursday. I will be with him when is confirm the cargo is unload."

"Is he going to Mexico to meet the ship when it arrives?"

"Maybe. He no tell me the plan after Thursday."

Rodríguez folded his note pad and put it back in his pocket, then looked at Vicente skeptically. "Vicente, if I get my people involved in this and you're lying about any of it, we'll come down on you so hard it will seem like paradise next to what you've been through."

"Ok, I understand," Vicente replied, but he doubted that anything the FBI or DEA could subject him to was worse than what he'd experienced in Fidel's prisons.

The agent stood and offered his hand. "I'm going against my better judgment here and trusting you on this," said Rodríguez. "Don't disappoint me."

Vicente laughed for a second and answered, "This the same thing everyone tell me, more or less. No to worry, I call you if the plan change."

Rodríguez allowed himself a brief smile before he turned and walked back towards downtown. Vicente shook his head and walked back to his car. Now that the task force was informed it was time to let Jim Morgan know about the sub. That would get him back in the good graces of his former controller and should earn him a favor in the future.

Vicente arrived back at the office after lunch and apparently after Rita had left. He thought she must have delayed her lunch to be at the phone in case Leslie Robertson called, because it was nearly two in the afternoon and she hadn't returned. On his desk he saw a message scribbled on a piece of paper from her note pad: call Leslie. He immediately dialed the RBDF office and the call rang through to Leslie's assistant, Dominica.

"Oh, yes, Mr. Amarón. How nice to hear from you. The Commander is away on a lunch break at the moment but I'll be sure to let him know you called."

"Thank you," he answered.

So the only thing left to do was to call Morgan in Langley. Vicente wasn't even certain he'd take the call, but it was worth a try. He searched around in his wallet until he found Morgan's business card. All it contained was his name, James Morgan, and a telephone number. It was typical of the types of cards Agency personnel gave out to assets or contacts. Nothing incriminating to suggest their affiliation, directing all calls onto a clean, secure line.

Vicente concentrated hard because he knew that Morgan disliked the fact the he couldn't speak English very well. He vowed to speak slowly and get the words right, at least as much as he could.

He waited while the phone rang at the other end. Three rings. Five rings. Eight rings and still no answer.

He was about to hang up when someone picked up at the other end.

"Yeah. Who is this?"

"I am Vicente Amarón. I call for Jim Morgan."

Initially there was only silence, then, "Hang on a minute."

The call went to hold for several minutes and Vicente contemplated how and what exactly he would tell Morgan about the whole affair. He quickly decided to tell him everything, as holding back might jeopardize Morgan's participation. Besides, he might need his help locating Eli if the RBDF hadn't been successful.

"This is Morgan. Who's this?"

"Vicente. How are you, Jim?"

"Just fine, Vicente. At least you used a secure line this time."

Vicente remembered how mad Morgan had been the last time he contacted him. He'd called the general number at the Langley office, the unsecured line The Agency used to conduct normal business and one that was frequently monitored by just about every other intelligence service in the world. Morgan was really hot about that breach of security.

"Jim, there is a problem. Eli is missing and I think maybe he has much trouble."

"Vicente, you know we're not a missin' persons service here. What else is on your mind?"

Morgan was characteristically impatient, but his attitude surprised Vicente a little. "Yes, Jim, you are correct. There is more. I want to tell you about a Russian submarine, OSKAR-1 Class, that comes to Cuba soon. It carry drugs for the Medellín Cartel."

Again there was silence at the other end of the line, then Morgan said, "Ok, go on. You've got my attention."

Vicente told him everything he'd just told Rodríguez, including the involvement of the Orchid task force.

Morgan was quiet while Vicente told his story. When he'd finished, Morgan said, "How the hell did you guys get mixed up in all this shit? Can't you stay outta' trouble for fifteen damn minutes without me checkin' on you?"

"Jim, this no our fault. So tell me, what we will do?"

"*We*?" said Morgan, incredulously. "*We* ain't doin' shit. You go ahead and finish what you started with the task force. We won't piss in their pool. I guess I'll have to call the DOD so they can alert the Coast Guard. Maybe we can catch 'em when they get back into Colombian territorial waters." He paused again and added, "That was good information, Vicente. So what do you want in return?"

Vicente nodded and replied, "You know me very well, Jim. Yes, there are two thing. First, I need help to find Eli and get him back to Miami. You must promise and send me whatever I need. Next, the Coast Guard must know the tip come from Eli. Can you do this?"

"Yep, I can do both of those things," said Morgan. "Call me when you have him located and we'll set everythin' up. I'll see what I can do with Defense, but they're pretty hard to deal with on these types of things."

"Thank you, Jim. I know you do you best. I call

when we locate Eli."

"Before you go," added Morgan. "I may have another contract for you soon. Talk to Eli for me when he gets back, see if he's interested."

"I will. Goodbye." Vicente hung up and smiled. At least he would be able to get Eli back to Miami. He just needed to find him first. He suddenly heard the door open and the familiar sound of Rita's keys jingling on her keychain.

"Rita, please to call back Leslie for me?"

"Sure, honey," she called out from her desk.

A few minutes passed before Rita rang his phone. "I have Leslie Robertson on the line," she said. "I'll connect you."

Vicente's phone rang and he said, "Leslie, what you know now? Where is Eli and Jo McHenry?"

"Vicente, we've looked everywhere for them and cannot find them. But Perry Barnes at AUTEC phoned me on Monday evening and confirmed that they left Andros Town on Sunday morning, so that means they went missing yesterday. We also know that a private jet took off from Norman's Cay yesterday afternoon with no flight plan on file. Maybe they were on that plane. I'm sorry, but that's the best we can do."

"I understand. Thank you, Leslie. Please to keep looking. I tell you if Eli contact me."

He hung up, disappointed but not disheartened. Vicente knew that Eli and Jo were Ok as recently as yesterday morning, and he was confident that Eli would find a way to get himself and Jo out of whatever trouble they were in. He just needed to be ready to act when he got the word. He only hoped it would be before Thursday.

Chapter 20

"You are impressed?" asked Manuel, smiling at Eli.

The *pirogue* bounced in the waves so Eli allowed his head to nod in rhythm.

"You guys are very resourceful. That will make my job a lot easier. So when can we leave? We won't have much time to get back, get a boat and meet your teams."

"This shipment is bound for Cuba, so maybe next time. For now you will be my guests in Mount Harris. It's been a long time since I've had such interesting and beautiful company." He stared at Jo, who smiled weakly and then stared ahead at the oncoming beach.

"But that wasn't the deal, Manuel. You said your routes were compromised." Eli could sense something was wrong, as Manuel's attitude had changed after his call to Miami.

"You are the one who said that," Manuel shot back. "You are the one trying to throw doubt into the equation, telling me my people in Miami are disloyal. I don't believe this.....yet. So the deal is whatever I say it is. You will stay with me until the cargo makes it safely to Cuba. Then we'll see what we do about you." The smile was gone and his expression was now deadly serious.

"Cuba? You're sending the sub to Cuba? How the hell does that work?"

The boat slowed for its approach to the beach and the mate ran forward to pull it in.

Manuel turned to Eli and answered, "Sorry, I forgot to mention that part. If this experiment works out, we will have a new transshipment point. Then we won't need to use the Bahamas any longer."

He walked forward to exit the boat and added, "We'll see if you are still useful on Friday." Manuel climbed down the ladder to the sand with Jo right behind.

The mate helped her down and Eli joined her, jumping directly down from the boat. He and Jo followed Manuel up the path to the waiting Land Rovers and headed for separate vehicles as before, but Arthur bowed his head slightly so Eli grabbed Jo by the hand.

"Ride with me," he said quietly.

"Miss McHenry, where are you going?" Manuel called out.

"She wants to talk to me for awhile," said Eli. "Be nice and share."

"As you wish." Manuel got into the middle vehicle and Eli and Jo got into the third one, displacing one of the guards. One guy just shrugged and went up to join his boss, while the other guy occupied the front passenger's seat next to Arthur.

"Welcome back, Eli," said Arthur.

"Sure Arthur. Good to be here. Drive safely."

"Oh, no problem wit dat one." He waited for the other Rovers to pull out and then fell in behind them, the last vehicle in the caravan.

"So why did you want me to ride with you?" said Jo.

"I was lonely," lied Eli. Arthur chuckled to himself. "Besides, I still want to know what you agreed to with the big boss."

Jo sighed dramatically. "As I said before, my business is *my* business, and I will keep some things to myself when I choose."

"And this is one of those things?"

"Yes," was her curt reply.

Eli could only assume from her answer that Jo had made the proverbial deal with the devil to get the financing she needed. He wondered what else she'd promised Manuel to maybe "sweeten" the deal. No matter, as they would be traveling for a couple of hours down the winding two-lane road back to Mount Harris.

Jo fell asleep after the first half hour and her head rested on Eli's shoulder. The heavily shrouded road eventually gave way to the open views of the coast, and then they were headed inland again towards Sangre Grande. He could see Arthur checking the rear view mirror every half hour to see if they were both sleeping, but Eli forced himself to stay awake and observant. He knew something was in the works, but not what and when it might happen.

Eli looked down at Jo, her platinum hair twisted into a tight bun and still smelling of flowers from her shampoo. He allowed himself to wonder what it would be like to be with one person permanently, to *feel* that way about one person. He thought about the women in his life who'd meant something to him in the last few years.

There were really only two. Violeta was one, and while he cared for her when he was in self-imposed exile in Costa Rica, he never felt committed to her. That was because he always knew he'd go back to his old job one day, and that meant eventually having to leave. And Mai Lee was the other. She took his breath away, but he knew they existed in totally different worlds that just came together by chance for awhile. He rationalized away his lack of commitment to her by making himself believe it was in her best interest for him to leave. *Was I just kidding myself?* he wondered.

Now there was Jo, the soon to be rich socialite with enough brass and attitude to stand up to him, yet a girl that also seemed to be vulnerable on so many levels. Could he ever hope to dream of capturing someone like her? Or would that turn out to be just as much of an illusion as his other relationships had been? Eli wasn't sure, but for the short term he wasn't going to let himself focus on anything else but getting out of Trinidad.

He began to grow tense after they'd passed through Sangre Grande and were once again headed south to the compound at Mount Harris. He noticed Arthur was now checking his mirror frequently, and appeared nervous.

"Arthur, you feeling Ok?" asked Eli.

"Yeah, boss. We doin' fine."

Arthur was less than convincing, and Eli expected

that whatever was going to happen would start when they arrived at the compound. He put his hand on Jo's cheek and whispered, "Jo, time to get up. We're almost there."

Her eyes popped open and she straightened in her seat, trying to get her bearings. "Sorry I fell asleep on you," she said with a yawn.

"No worries. But you need to stay awake now. Something doesn't feel right to me, and I think there's going to be trouble."

"Trouble? What sort of trouble?"

"I don't know exactly. But if something happens, I want you to stay close. We may need to make a run for it." Eli looked into her eyes to make sure she saw he was serious. She nodded and bit her lip.

The caravan turned off the road and approached the gate to Manuel's jungle "resort," and the guard in the front vehicle got out to unlock it and usher them through. As the Rovers arrived at the house Eli could see that the lights were off, and instantly realized they were in trouble.

"Stick with me," he said to Jo.

The guards got out of the first vehicle and approached the house. Manuel got out and shouted for Julio, but no one answered. The guard in Eli's car, seeing that something was wrong, drew a pistol from his shoulder holster and had one hand on the door when Arthur reached over with his right hand and shoved a Glock 17 against his head and pulled the trigger.

Eli saw it coming and covered Jo with his body, forcing her to the floor of the Rover. The guard's head exploded against the side window as the bullet exited the car, and he slumped over and fell out the partially opened door.

"Stay down!" shouted Arthur to his passengers.

He leaped out of the Rover and began firing at Manuel and the other Colombians. Just at that moment, gunfire erupted from all sides of them and a large Jeep came screaming into the drive just behind them. Three guys with MAC-10's started firing at the cars, while eight other guys emerged from the bushes around the house. Bullets rained down on the Colombians, who were caught out in the open with no place to take cover.

It was all over in less than a minute. Six bodyguards and the other two drivers were dead, crumpled in odd positions on the ground, some in the vehicles. Manuel lay on the ground close to the house.

Eli stuck his head up and opened the door to get out.

"Don't move!" he shouted at Jo, and then he went over to Arthur. The other men immediately pointed their weapons at Eli but Arthur quickly intervened.

"He Ok," Arthur shouted. "He wit me now. Clean de place, boys! Move ahead wit de plan!"

Arthur nodded to Eli, who then knelt down by Manuel. He'd been shot through the chest at least once and was lying face down, gasping for air. Eli rolled him over and propped his back up against his knee as Jo walked over slowly with a horrified look on her face.

"Bad luck, Manuel," said Eli.

"Is the nature of the business," he replied hoarsely. "So you were right after all. I guess I should have listened to you."

"Yes, but you can't go back and do it again."

"No, you are right. Please take care of the lady."

"You can count on it," Eli answered. Manuel lifted his hand weakly and waved at him.

Arthur walked over and said to Eli, "Put he down now. Is over fuh he."

Eli laid Manuel down carefully and the dying drug lord coughed up a lung full of foamy blood. He went over and pulled Jo away, back towards the Rover as Arthur passed him.

Arthur pointed the Glock at Manuel's head and said, "Nothin' personal, boss man," then pulled the trigger.

Jo shrieked and jumped at the sound, and cowered as Eli escorted her back to the rear passenger seat of their Rover.

"Stay here," Eli said quietly but firmly.

The other gunmen began pulling the bodies from the lawn and the vehicles into the house. Arthur came with a towel from one of the bathrooms and cleaned up the seat and window next to him, then threw it into the house. The rest of his gang ransacked the place in search of anything valuable and then pulled the other Rovers away from the building.

"Get in," said Arthur forcefully, and he drove them recklessly out towards the Cunapo Southern Road.

Eli looked over his shoulder and saw that the house was on fire, and the other two Rovers and the Jeep were racing up from behind. Jo shivered next to him and he put his arm around her to try and comfort her. She began to sob hysterically and all Eli could do was pat her head and whisper, "It's Ok. We're Ok."

The Rover burst out onto the road without stopping, as if no other vehicles ever travelled that way. They swerved and skidded until Arthur regained control and then they shot north towards Sangre Grande. The Rover's engine screamed and protested at being driven that hard, but soon they were a mile from the turn off and the horrific scene at the compound. The other vehicles turned abruptly south and headed towards the town of Biche. Eli guessed they would head into the Central Range soon and would dump the Rovers where no one would find them, then be on their way as if nothing had happened.

Arthur looked in his mirror to see how his "passengers" were doing. "Yuh doin' Ok back der?"

Eli sat up so that Arthur could see him clearly. "Not bad, considering what just happened. So what's the plan for us? Do we get the same as Manuel and his boys?"

Arthur laughed his low, rumbling laugh and slapped the steering wheel. He slowed down and stared at Eli with his off eye. "Cool yuhself, Eli. Yuh two not part uh de deal," he answered.

"What deal?"

"Duh worry 'bout dat."

"Arthur, I'm not trying to push. No way I want to do that," said Eli softly. "But I'm sure you can guess what we're thinking right now."

Arthur smiled and nodded. "Duh worry, bredda. We no gone harm yuh. Dis were payback for whut dem Colombians done ah mih boys in the Bahamas last week." He spit into the passenger's seat for emphasis and then paused to contemplate the situation a bit more.

"Ah need some time tuh tink 'bout dis. Yuh wit me now, least 'till we get tuh Port a Spain. So relax an hold yuh gyul." He refocused on the road and drove on at a more reasonable pace.

Jo managed to get control of herself and she sat up straight in the back seat. She wiped the tears from her face and said to Eli, "What happens next?"

"That all depends on our friend Arthur here."

Arthur waved at Jo and smiled.

"Eli, I have to get back to Miami. They're going to have the Board meeting next week and I have to prepare everything."

"Doh worry Miss Jo," said Arthur. "Yuh get back some time."

Jo looked at Eli, who just shrugged.

They all sat silently until they were back on the eastern Main Road and clear of Sangre Grande. Eli decided to probe again to see if he could find out who was behind what had happened at the compound.

"So Arthur, you working for the Cali Cartel? Did they order the hit on Manuel and his operation? Or is this something else?"

"Der yuh go again, actin' like a maco. But ah guess is no trouble tuh tell yuh whut goin' down." He looked into the mirror to make sure Eli was paying attention.

"Yuh see, is goin' like dis: Shower Posse got uh deal here, an dey doh like it when deez cocks move in tuh de neighborhood. De Colombians, man dey tink dey can buy everyone but yuh know whut? Dey wuz wrong."

"So you guys are Shower Posse?"

"We? Nah, but we all Caribbean breddas, an mih

boys can work wit dem Jamaicans. Ah wuz one year workin' tuh set dis plan in motion, but dat ting in de Bahamas was whut tip it over de edge. So today were yuh lucky day, Eli. Yuh got tuh see de results ah all mih hard work an planning." Arthur smiled.

"Now we clean up de house uh de rats an de world be a good place again."

Eli nodded in agreement. "I get it. You couldn't let those guys move in unopposed and set up a permanent operation for fear of losing control of your own turf. Makes sense to me. But why didn't you just kill us back there in the forest?" Jo poked Eli hard in the shoulder and shot him a dirty look.

"Cuz ah can see yuh not one uh dem, Eli, nor yuh lady der. Dat wuz clear from de start. Who yuh be an why yuh here, ah doh know. But ah tink maybe yuh got uh use. So whut yuh tink? Ah hole yuh fuh ransom? Whut ah get fuh yuh?"

Eli laughed nervously. "Well, you can't get much for me, but I can help you look good to the Jamaicans. Miss McHenry is a different story, as I'm sure you already know. But if you let us both go, I'll give you something better than a short term bump in pay."

Arthur turned so that his off eye looked straight at Eli while he drove.

"I can tell the Jamaicans where and how the Colombians are bringing their dope into Trinidad. You can arrange to grab a shipment and then it's all yours."

"Very interesting. Leh mih tink 'bout it."

Their pace became more leisurely the farther they got from the compound, and Arthur began to hum to himself as they neared Port of Spain.

"Whut yuh tink, Eli? Ah should trust yuh or ah doh?"

"Oh, you should trust me, Arthur. Absolutely no question. I won't steer you wrong."

The big "Rasta" laughed again and said, "Yuh know whut? Ah feelin' lucky today. We goin' fuh a ride."

Eli thought he'd turn right off the highway and go into the labyrinth of streets south of town known as the Laventille district. The area was notorious as a home for criminal gangs and was as violent as any populated area in Cali or Medellín. But it was also one of the birth places of the "pan" orchestras, the popular steel drum bands that played during Carnival time in Trinidad. Eli had first heard the Amoco Renegades at a pan yard in Laventille, his introduction to the sophisticated and captivating music once traditionally produced from the heads of fifty-five gallon oil drums. So while he acknowledged the harsh reality of the district, he still appreciated what it had to offer, at least from a musical point of view.

Indeed, Arthur did turn off and the vehicle wound its way up into the neighborhood, row after row of houses and shops blighted by poverty and violence, and in sore need of government help. He went up towards Picton Quarry and then pulled over next to a rum shop.

"Stay here if yuh know whut good fuh yuh," Arthur said.

The presence of a new Land Rover was an attention grabber in Laventille, and the curious soon began to stare at the foreign couple in the back seat. Arthur thankfully wasn't gone for more than a couple of minutes, and he shot a dirty look at the small crowd that had gathered near the vehicle. They immediately dispersed and he got in and started driving again.

"Ah goin' tuh drop yuh at de Hilton. Best fuh yuh der. So now, Eli, yuh tell mih where I goin' find de Colombians."

Eli spoke while Arthur unraveled them from the neighborhood and drove north to Queens Park Savannah. Eli told him what he knew, about how the drugs traveled out from Punta Pescador via *pirogue* to a rendezvous at Manzanilla Point. He guessed there would be another shipment in two days, enough time to stockpile the drugs before the sub returned from Cuba. He suggested that a few fast boats masquerading as fisherman could intercept the *pirogues* coming into Trinidadian waters and hijack the cargoes without anyone being the wiser for it.

"Maybe ah wuz wrong 'bout yuh," said Arthur afterwards. "Yuh tink like mih boys. Sound like uh good plan. Maybe yuh want uh job wit we."

"No thanks. I've spent enough time trying to catch guys like you to want to join you now."

Jo elbowed Eli in the ribs but Arthur just laughed his big laugh.

"Dat why mih like yuh, Eli. Yuh uh honest man."

He laughed some more as the exhausted Rover turned up Lady Young Road and drove up the hill. Arthur was laughing so hard he almost missed the sharp left turn into the Hilton driveway. He cut the wheel hard, causing the oncoming vehicle to blow it's horn, but once in the parking area, he proceeded slowly to the front of the hotel.

The drivers from St. Christopher's taxi service gawked at Arthur as he drove up to the guest drop off. Eli thought some must have recognized him, but no one said anything audible. The bellman opened the passenger door and said, "Welcome, welcome. Just checking in?"

"Hey boy," shouted Arthur. "Yuh take care mih friends here, understand?"

The kid looked stunned but nodded his head as Jo and Eli exited the left side door.

"Good. Eli, ah got something fuh yuh." Eli leaned over the driver's door and Arthur thrust a note at him.

"Take it. Yuh come back here an need help one day, yuh call mih." He looked sincere and offered his huge hand.

Eli shook his hand enthusiastically and said, "Good luck, my friend, and be careful. Remember the old Trinidadian proverb: "What yuh do in de darkness mus' come to light."

The big guy laughed again and replied, "Ah goin' tuh see 'bout mih. Now is yuh tuh ketch." He drove through the roundabout and Eli could hear him laughing as the Rover disappeared back down the hill.

"What did that mean?" asked Jo.

"It means, I'm taken care of. Now you're on your own."

Chapter 21

Eli believed in miracles. Small ones, large ones, whatever. He'd had miraculous escapes from death a number of times over the years, events he often thought of as large miracles. They'd happened so often, what else could he think? And when he did walk into misfortune, he had still been the beneficiary of small miracles as well, like the one that brought Jo to his door. One thing they all had in common was that he never took any of those providential gifts for granted. Their escape alive and uninjured from Manuel's compound had been yet another example of a large miracle, but there was still one small miracle left he hadn't counted on.

Checking into a major hotel dirty and disheveled, without bags, money, or identification would have been impossible without such a miracle. And just when he most needed one, there it was.

On their way up to reception, Eli spied a familiar face at the concierge's desk. It was Harry Carleton, a senior manager for Amoco Trinidad Oil Company that he'd met at their Galeota Point facility many years earlier.

"Good grief, Harry!" exclaimed Eli with a smile. "I thought you would have retired by now."

"Hey, hey. Look what the cat dragged in! Eli, good ta' see ya'." Harry stood up and shook Eli's hand warmly. "And is this Mrs. Rose?" he said, smiling at Jo.

"Jo McHenry," she said, extending her hand. "No, we're just business partners, Mister?"

"Carleton. Harry Carelton. Nice ta' meet ya' Miss." His Oklahoma drawl was in full display and it reminded Eli of better times.

"Eli, ya' don't look so good. Everything Ok?"

Eli smiled at his tall friend. He'd lost all but a few strands of the strawberry blond hair that once topped his head, but he'd remained thin and looked to be in good health.

"Well, now that you mention it, we've had sort of a bad time today. We were out on the north coast to do some sightseeing and ran into some highway men. They got our wallets and passports, so we're kind of in a pickle."

Harry frowned and cursed. "Damn I hate ta' hear about crap like that. What can I do ta' help?" He pushed his glasses back over his forehead and looked at Jo with an expression of deep concern.

"We need a place to stay tonight and some clean clothes. Do you guys have any place up here where we can clean up and get some rest?"

Harry rubbed his thin hair and looked at the floor for a second. "No. We got rid of the apartments here, but I got some leverage with the hotel. Lemme' see what I can do." He looked a bit dated, with his knit Ralph Lauren polo shirt tucked into his high-riding trousers, but he was as resourceful a guy as Eli had ever met.

He walked over to one of the girls at reception and spoke with her for a few seconds. She disappeared back into the office and quickly returned with the hotel manager, who looked over at Eli and Jo as Harry explained their situation. They shook and hands and the manager smiled and waved at the couple across the way.

Eli and Jo waved back and Harry motioned for them to come over.

"Please fill out these registration cards down to here," said the girl, pointing at the home address line. They each grabbed a pen and began to write as Harry explained.

"You'll stay tonight as my guests. Whatever ya' need from the boutique or anywhere in town, ya' can charge it ta' me. We can't let things like this happen ta' our visitors, now can we, Doreen?"

Doreen smiled while she entered their information into the hotel's computer system.

"Harry, you know I'm good for it. I'll make it up to you right away," said Eli, shaking his hand again.

"Nonsense. Don't worry. You all just get ta' your room and relax. I'm just glad ta' be of help."

"You're a prince, old friend," said Eli.

"Yes, an absolute life saver. Thanks so much," added Jo, who stood on her toes to kiss him on the cheek.

"Well, that's worth it right there," laughed Harry.

Doreen handed the keys to Jo and said, "Take the elevator at the far end, then down to three."

Jo smiled and looked at her curiously. "*Down* to three?"

"I'll explain," said Eli, getting up. "Look, Harry. I'll call you tomorrow and let you know what arrangements we've made. I'm expecting that we might make one of the Miami flights if we're lucky, so I'll send you a check."

"Forget it, Eli," Harry replied. "Next time I'm in Miami ya' can wine and dine me around town. Jo, it was a pleasure ta' meet ya'." Harry shook her hand. "Ya'll get some rest and try and enjoy the rest of your time here. Again I'm sorry ta' hear about what happened to ya.' Sorry I can't stay, but I've got a dinner with one of my guys from Houston. Gotta' go." They shook hands again and Harry left, loping stiffly down the walk to the entrance.

Eli looked at the keys in Jo's hand and said, "Follow me."

He walked towards the back of the lobby and opened the glass doors to the walkway to the new part of the hotel. The setting sun shone brightly off the waters of the Gulf of Paria and presented a spectacular view from the veranda. They walked down the teak and mahogany hallway that led to the second elevator bank and then Eli said, "Watch this." They were on the Lobby level and to get to the third floor, he pressed the "down" elevator button.

"Why on earth did you do that?" asked Jo. "We're on the third floor, not the basement."

"You've never heard of the famous "Upside Down

Hilton" I take it?"

"What?"

"Ok, I'll explain how it works. You might not have noticed as we were driving up, but the hotel is built on the side of a hill. Instead of going up the hill, they constructed the rooms going down the hill, so the higher floors are actually farther *down* the hill than the lobby. It takes a bit of getting used to but it works."

The elevator opened and Eli said, "Push three and see what happens."

Jo pushed the button and the elevator went down, just as he said it would. "Wow, that's really strange, but kind of fun" she said.

They exited on three and went down the carpet-lined hallway to their room.

"Eli, before I get cleaned up I need some clean clothes to change into. I'm going *up* to the boutique to get a few essentials."

"Sounds like a plan. I'll do the same."

They went back up to the lobby and down the hall to the boutique, which was located in one of the small shops that lined the attached shopping promenade. Jo bought a couple of light-weight dresses and blouses, along with a pair of open-toed shoes and an assortment of undergarments, while Eli picked up a new shirt and trousers for himself. They walked next door to the small pharmacy and purchased toothbrushes, combs, and other toiletries and then walked back to the room.

"You first," he said, offering Jo the shower.

"You won't have to ask me twice." She went into the bathroom and soon, Eli heard her singing in the shower.

He picked up the phone and said, "I need to place a call to the US." He gave the operator the number and put the receiver down for a second so she could ring back with the call.

"Brickell Avenue Associates. This is Rita speaking."

"Rita, it's Eli. I..........." was all he could get out before Rita burst out in tears.

"Eli, thank God you're Ok. We've been worried sick about you. We thought you were dead, I was so worried, I didn't know what to think. I..........."

"Rita," Eli shouted into the receiver. "Calm down. Everything's Ok. I need to talk to Vicente right now. Is he in the office?"

"Yes, sure. Just a moment."

The phone clicked over to the canned music that played for callers on hold, a set of "Easy Listening" tunes that Rita chose because she liked Barry Manilow. Eli rolled his eyes while he waited.

"Eli, is really you?" said Vicente.

"Is really me, old friend. Listen, I've got to pass along some intel really quick before I lose my chance. Jo and I were brought to Trinidad by Manuel Durán, one of Pablo Escobar's "expediters" for the Caribbean. They are sending a large shipment of coke north via a base somewhere in Cuba and they're using a decommissioned Russian nuclear sub to do it. You've got to notify the Coast Guard and maybe Jim Morgan of what's going on."

"Eli, I already do this. I know about the submarine. Thanks to God you and Jo are Ok. I go to call Jim so he send a plane for you both tomorrow. We have many more thing to discuss."

"I know, but I don't have much time. Listen, we also pretty much confirmed that Jo's parents are dead, likely murdered by the Shower Posse. They were probably in the wrong place at the wrong time."

"I was think that maybe this is so. I sorry to hear this. She is Ok?"

"She seems to be, but you're right that we have a lot more to discuss."

Vicente sighed. "Ok, Eli. Jim calls you tomorrow to say when he come to get you and Jo. I see you in the office on Wednesday."

"Bye old friend."

Eli hung up the phone just as the shower stopped running. He opened the sliding glass door and went out to sit on the balcony. The view looked across the Queen's Park Savannah, where a soccer match was playing out in the waning hours of the afternoon sun. The shadows were stretched out long across the city and small *troupial* birds flitted in and out of the trees that lined the hillside below. Eli lost himself for a moment in the serenity of scene, letting his thoughts drift for the first time since Miami.

"All yours," said Jo as she opened the steamy bathroom door. She wore one of the white hotel robes that hung in the bathroom and dried her hair with a towel.

"God, it feels so good to get really clean."

"I hope to find out," Eli said. "Please excuse me."

She smiled and took his seat on the balcony while he showered.

The hot water felt restorative and soothed his aching muscles. Feeling clean again also made him feel better able to deal with whatever Morgan would throw at him. He almost looked forward to seeing his old handler again, especially since he was rescuing him from some dire circumstances. But he also knew there would be a price to pay for a special plane, the crew, and the agents that Morgan would send for him. That part was not going to be fun. But at least for now he could relax and let someone else worry about how to get them out of Trinidad and back into the US.

"You getting hungry?" said Eli as he stood in the hallway, clad in the other hotel robe.

Jo had a towel wrapped around her head, turban-style, and her feet rested on the balcony railing. "I'm famished. I could eat a horse."

"Well, the restaurant here is pretty good from what I remember. I'm afraid we don't have any other choice on this little "visit" as I'm presently a bit strapped for cash, but if we ever get back here I'll take you to a really good Indian place I've heard good things about."

"Sounds yummy," she said with a smile. "But it's still a bit early for dinner here, isn't it?"

Eli looked at his watch. "Yeah, but we should be Ok in an hour or so."

Jo stretched out on the bed and propped herself up on her elbows. "So, what can we do for the next hour, I wonder?" She smiled and opened her robe at the waist, revealing her long, muscular legs up to her beautiful blond triangle.

"Got any ideas?"

Eli couldn't believe his good fortune. He said, "Save

that thought," and quickly hung the "Do not disturb" sign on the door.

"I think you're happy to see me again," she purred, noting the conspicuous and rapidly growing bulge under his robe.

"How could you tell?" he said as he laid down beside her.

"Oh, I don't know. Woman's intuition."

"What about dinner?"

"It can wait."

§

"You get it, I'm not ready to talk to anyone." Jo rolled over and punched Eli in the arm so he would get up and answer the phone.

"Yes, this is Mr. Rose. Who's this?"

"John Holcomb, US Embassy. I received a call this morning from Washington requesting me to issue new US passports to you and a Miss Josephine McHenry. I'm going to send a car for you in thirty minutes, if that's Ok."

"Yeah, sure, that's fine. We'll be ready. Thanks." Eli pulled the pillow off Jo's head and said, "That was the embassy. They're going to issue us new passports, but we've got to get going. The car will be here in a half hour."

Jo rolled over on her side and said, "I'm too tired. You go without me."

"Sorry, boss. Time for us to head home. You want the bathroom first?"

"I'm going, I'm going."

She got up slowly and stretched at the foot of the bed, her lithe body lit only by the sun that filtered in through the gap in the curtain that covered the sliding glass door. The sight woke Eli up and he stared at her nude form as she walked off to the bathroom.

"What are you staring at?" she said, knowing full well what the answer was.

"The most amazing looking girl I've ever seen."

"Well, don't get too used to it. We won't be doing this when we're back in Miami."

Eli was floored and his expression evidently reflected it.

"Oh, don't look like that," she added. "We can still have fun. Just not as publically as here."

She closed the door and Eli rolled over on his back to try and comprehend what she'd just said. *I guess she would be embarrassed by me,* he thought. *I'm not from the right social class, or something.* He got up and quickly pulled his clothes on before she came back into the room.

"Your turn," she said with a smile.

Eli went in to wash his face and brush his teeth. *She's not at all concerned with how I took that. I must have made way too much of this whole thing.* He felt foolish for falling for her, and he was mad at himself for letting the fantasy of a meaningful relationship creep into his brain. *Gotta' snap out of this,* he thought. *It's no big deal for her, so it shouldn't be any big deal for me, either.*

"I'll buy you a late breakfast or an early lunch when we get back from the embassy, "Eli called out. *From now on it's just business,* he told himself.

"Ok, I'm ready. You ready to go?"

"Ready to go," she answered in a cheery voice. Jo smiled brightly and looked much younger in her sleeveless, island-style sun dress. She had her hair pinned up in a ponytail like a teenager and she reached out to hold his arm as they walked to the elevator.

Eli was uncertain if she wanted to maintain their casual relationship or if she'd already slipped into one that was more formal. They went down to the hotel entrance and sat on one of the wooden benches to wait for the embassy car.

A black Chevy Suburban soon pulled up and a young guy wearing a dark coat and sunglasses got out of the passengers side and approached Eli.

"Are you Mr. Rose?"

"Yes, Are you Mr. Holcomb?"

"Yes. Please come with me." He opened the driver's side rear door and the bellman ran around to open the other door. Jo and Eli got in and Holcomb got into the front seat. He shook Eli's hand first, then Jo's.

"John Holcomb. Good to meet you. So, I understand you both have had a pretty difficult time here."

Jo looked at Eli for guidance, so Eli said, "Well, it's not been a traditional vacation, if that's what you mean."

Holcomb smiled. "Sorry about that. These types of robberies are becoming a more serious problem than in years past, that's for sure. It can be more than a little upsetting from what everyone tells me."

"It certainly was," said Jo, playing into the deception.

"Well, don't worry. We'll have some new passports

for you today. We just need to take your photos and get some basic information from you first."

He's being inordinately polite, thought Eli. *I wonder what's up?*

Holcomb pulled off his sunglasses and swept a lock of long, black hair from his eyes.

"We'll have you on your way by this evening."

"That's pretty quick," said Eli. "By the way, you wouldn't happen to have any messages for me, would you?"

"Now that you mention it, yes," said Holcomb in a near whisper. "But I'll have to tell you when we arrive at the embassy." He passed a sideways look over at the driver, intending to send the message that he did not trust him enough to deliver the message in his presence.

"That's fine. Whatever you want," Eli replied. "Is the embassy still over on Marli Street?"

"Yes, it is, but we really need a new space. So you've visited us before?"

"Yes."

"When was that?"

"Probably when you were about nine years old," said Eli, tiring of Holcomb's small talk.

"Oh, I see," said the young consular officer. "Yes, that would have been around 1972, a bit before my time I'm afraid. Well, you didn't miss anything. Trinidad's been pretty much the same since then."

Eli saw the driver working hard not to smile.

"Mr. Holcomb, is this your first overseas posting?" said Jo.

"Yes, it is. Does it show?"

Jo and Eli both smiled. "No, not at all. It's just that

you're really enthusiastic about your job," said Jo in a sympathetic voice. "That's a good thing where I come from."

He smiled and said, "Thanks. It's nice of you to say." He turned around and faced the front of the vehicle, apparently content that he'd made a good first impression.

The Suburban pulled around to the employees entrance and the guards stopped them at the gate. The driver showed his ID and reached over for Holcomb's as well. The guard handed the ID's back to the driver and waved for the other guard to open the gate. They drove in and Holcomb said, "Thank you, Robert. Mr. Rose, Miss McHenry, please follow me."

They thanked the driver and followed Holcomb through the security door and into the rear of the building. They walked up the stairs and he pointed them to a small conference room.

"Would you wait here please for a minute?"

"Sure," said Eli, and he and Jo sat down in the lightly padded chairs.

"Can I have my secretary bring you a coffee or some tea?"

"Coffee would be great," said Jo. "Black, no sugar."

"Some water would be nice," added Eli. Holcomb nodded and disappeared down the hall. His secretary returned a few moments later with the drinks. She placed them on the table and smiled. "Do yuh need anything else?"

"No, thanks, that's great," said Eli. She left and Jo gave Eli a funny look.

"What?"

"He's a little eager, don't you think" asked Jo, sipping her coffee.

"Holy cow, you think he's *a little eager*? If he was any more *eager* he'd be humping your leg like a Chihuahua."

Jo laughed suddenly, almost causing the coffee to shoot out of her nose.

Just at that moment, the *eager* consular officer returned and asked Jo to accompany him to his office.

"We can take your photo first and then get you to fill out the forms," he said with a smile.

She looked at Eli, still trying to stifle a laugh and swallow her coffee. She got up and with a wave and a smile at Eli, followed Holcomb out the door.

Eli smiled to himself but mere seconds later was greeted by a tired-looking Jim Morgan, wearing a slightly disheveled khaki coat, white shirt, and khaki trousers. He sported a particularly heavy five o'clock shadow, which was unlike the man. He looked tired but serious, and Eli knew this trip was not just a friendly gesture.

"Well, look what the cat coughed up," said Eli, shaking Morgan's hand. "It's been a long time, Jim. You're looking old and beat."

"Great to see you too, Eli. I'm lookin' like this 'cause I flew all damn night to get here. I came to pick you up and take you back to Miami."

"You personally came all this way in an Agency jet at this expense just for me? Come on, Jim, you know me better than that. Why are you really here?" Eli stared at his old handler, not really expecting to hear the truth.

Morgan smiled and stroked his thin hair. "Ok, Eli, no bullshit. I did come here to pick up you and the girl, but I also came because I needed to have a chat with my counterpart in the SIA. Care to come along for the ride?"

"What about Jo?"

"Oh, I'm sure our Mr. Holcomb will keep her occupied filling out forms and taking pictures for a couple of hours. This shouldn't take long."

"Sure, why not? For old times." said Eli.

"Yeah, for old times," said Morgan with a smile.

As they walked down to the car, Morgan handed Eli a newly minted US passport and added, "Courtesy of Uncle Sam. No thanks necessary."

They left through the back entrance to the building and took an embassy car over to the Red House, the building that housed Trinidad and Tobago's parliament. The nearly ninety year old red plaster and block building had a reputation for being steamy in the summer months, but it was fairly close to the embassy and an easier location for impromptu meetings of this type. Geoffrey Lin, Morgan's contact with the Security Intelligence Agency had requested they meet there, rather than at his office, as he had a meeting later in the day with the Prime Minister and it was more convenient for him.

Their driver went around to the back entrance, presented the two men's passports at the guard station and said, "Meeting with Mr. Lin." A quick call was made to verify the names and the meeting, and they were admitted to the building. Another guard escorted them to a side office on the first floor, where Lin was working at a small desk.

He smiled when he saw Morgan and stood to greet them. "Jim, good to see you again."

"Same, Geoffrey. Let me introduce Eli Rose. Eli is one of my best men." Morgan smiled at Eli, who was surprised by his introduction.

"A pleasure to meet you, Eli. Please sit down. I am just finishing up some materials that I need to show the PM when Parliament takes their morning break." Lin sat back and folded his hands over his chest.

"I got your message. What's so urgent that you had to personally fly here to tell me?"

Morgan's smile disappeared, giving way to a serious, almost pained expression.

"Geoffrey, we've been receivin' a lot of chatter recently that we don't normally hear, mostly between Port of Spain and various cities in the States, includin' my areas of jurisdiction in South Florida. Our sources tell us that somethin' big is in the works with Jamaat al-Muslimeen, and you should increase your surveillance efforts and keep a close wrap on them."

Lin nodded and listened intently while Morgan continued.

"We know they've been tryin' to purchase weapons and explosives in Florida and I believe they intend to use them here, against your government."

The balding agent adjusted his glasses and stroked his thin mustache nervously. Beads of sweat formed on his nearly bald head and he looked uncomfortable.

"That's very interesting news, Jim. Of course we've been monitoring their activities for some time now, but we have no indications that they are up to something. What makes you think an action is imminent?"

"The frequency of communications has increased a great deal over the past few months. As of the first of June the messages have gotten more specific and are usin' words like "plans" and "coordination." All I'm tellin' you is it doesn't smell right to me."

"I see," said Lin, introspectively. "And what would you suggest I do about this? At this point, they've broken no laws here in Trinidad and I cannot just detain them on suspicion of...........suspicion of just what, exactly? Can you connect any specific members with illegal acts in the United States?"

Morgan appeared frustrated but kept his cool.

"No, not at this point. But we'll round 'em up as soon as we think we have somethin' we can hold 'em on. Geoffrey, I'm just tryin' to return a favor. If you don't wanna' listen, that's fine with me. Just be advised that you've been warned. I've got a meetin' with the head of security over at Amoco and I'll be advisin' him to step up security at the Tatil buildin' and at Galeota Point. Just lettin' you know."

"Well, don't think I don't appreciate your efforts," said Lin. He uncrossed his hands and replaced them on the desk.

"I know you wouldn't have come unless you felt this was of critical importance. I'll take your suggestions under advisement and discuss your concerns with the PM. It's ultimately his call in matters of national security."

He got up to say goodbye, and shook hands again with his guests. "You must come back during Carnival next time, Jim. I'll show you a good time."

"I'll try and do that. Good to see you, Geoffrey, and good luck with everythin'."

"Good to meet you, Mr. Lin," said Eli.

"Ok, gentlemen. Take care." Lin sat back down and continued to shuffle through the papers on his desk as if he hadn't been interrupted. Morgan and Eli returned with their escort to the car, and they were passed through the gate without delay.

"Tatil Building," said Morgan to the driver. "Shit, that didn't go the way I'd hoped," he added quietly.

It was only a five minute trip over to the head office of the oil company, which was located in the twelve story Tatil Building on Maraval Road. It had been the tallest building in Port of Spain since its construction in 1974, but had recently been surpassed by the Central Bank and Eric Williams Finance buildings. It was aging, inside and out, and not gracefully.

The driver stopped on the street in front of the building and said, "Ah will park an come back tuh meet yuh here, suh."

"That's fine," said Morgan as he got out. "Let's go," he said to Eli, and the two men went into the building and to the guard's station.

"We have an appointment with Mr. Reilly," Morgan told the guard.

"Do yuh know de floor?" he answered.

"Yes."

"Den yuh can go up."

Morgan smiled thinly and led Eli to the elevator. When they arrived they were met by a secretary who ushered them into a conference room and offered them water or coffee. The men declined and sat silently, waiting for their host.

Fred Reilly was a impressive figure in person, an ex-Naval Intelligence officer who had retired after his twentieth year and jumped into the corporate world. His six foot five inch frame presented the image of a rough, heavy-handed individual, but it truth he was as even tempered and calm as could be.

"Jim, what brings you to these parts?" asked Reilly, shaking Morgan's hand.

"I'm in town on other business and I thought I'd stop by, in an unofficial capacity."

"Good, good. Well, good to see you again. And you are?"

"Eli Rose. I work with Jim from time to time." Eli smiled but Reilly didn't return the gesture.

"So what's on your mind, Jim?" Reilly sat back and slid his long legs under the table, away from his guests.

"Fred, we've been receivin' some intel in some of our offices about some type activity being planned here by Jamaat al-Muslimeen. I think they are gonna' strike at a high profile target somewhere in Trinidad within the next month. I just thought you should know."

"That's troubling," said Reilly, rubbing his gray temples with his fingers. "How confident are you of the source of the intel?"

"Very confident," replied Morgan with a sigh. "I think these guys have the motive and the resources in place to do some serious damage. You may want to increase security at your installations."

"Have you talked with Geoff Lin about this?"

"We just came from a meeting with him at the Red House, but he didn't seem too concerned about it. He seems to think they've got them well monitored and under control."

Reilly shook his head. "Sometimes that guy doesn't know his ass from a hole in the ground. I'll make the arrangements today. We'll put on some extra security and take some counter measures for the next forty-five days. If something's going to happen it should show up by then. You think there's any need to set up an evacuation plan?"

Morgan finally looked pleased. "No, not at this time. But I would have a list of all non-essential personnel and plans in place to move them, just in case the lid blows off this place."

"Ok, sounds like a prudent plan. Anything else?"

"That's it. I hope I was of some help."

"My door is always open," said Reilly, standing "I'll walk you out." They walked to the elevators and he added, "Sorry I don't have more time for you today but I have a review with management later that I need to get ready."

"No worries," said Morgan. "Maybe I'll have Eli come down in a few weeks with an update, if we have one." Eli stared at him but Morgan pretended not to notice.

"Let me know if your people hear anythin' that might be useful."

"Will do," said Reilly. "Have a good trip back." They shook hands and got on the elevator.

"Since when am I your messenger boy?" said Eli as they rode down.

"Just tryin' to be helpful," Morgan replied. "Besides, you never know. I might even have a little job for you when you get back."

Eli said nothing, not wanting to seem ungrateful for his rescue. But he had no intention of working for The Agency again once he had Jo back in Miami. They reached the ground floor and left the building to meet their driver, who was waiting by the entrance.

"Stay here, suh. I come get yuh wit de car." The guy ran off and Morgan looked up towards the eastern sky.

"Eli, I think a storm is coming, and I don't necessarily mean the weather."

"I know. When can we get out of here?"

"We'll go collect your Miss McHenry and I'll take you back to the Hilton so you can pack your things. I'd like to be in the air by three at the latest."

The car arrived and they jumped in the back seat. They arrived back at the embassy just as it began to rain, slowly at first and then in a constant, heavy curtain. Eli and Morgan returned to the conference room and in a few minutes Holcomb appeared with Jo trailing behind.

"You must be the lovely Miss McHenry," said Morgan, standing to greet her. "My name is Jim Morgan. I'm an old friend of Eli's, and I've come here to take you back to Miami."

Jo smiled broadly and shook his hand. "Well I am sure glad to see you, Mr. Morgan. Please call me Jo."

"Eli, you ready?" Morgan looked at him expectantly.

"Yes, you bet," replied Eli. "Mr. Holcomb, thanks for all your help. We really appreciate it."

"Oh, you're most welcome. Miss McHenry, it was a pleasure to meet you." Holcomb shook her hand limply and Jo could only smile.

"I'm having lunch with the ambassador, so I'll mention your help. Thanks again." Morgan shook his hand as well.

"Yes, sir. Anything I can ever do to help, you can count on me." Holcomb stood straight as a pole and Eli thought he might even salute Morgan.

Morgan just smiled thinly and the group went back down to the waiting Suburban.

The rain had stopped and the sun was shining through the great clouds of steam that rose from the drenched asphalt of the parking area. They drove back around the Savannah, through the roundabout at Lady Young Road and on to the Hilton.

"I'll pick you up no later than two this afternoon," said Morgan as they reached the entrance. "I've already transferred the charges for your stay to my account, so feel free to check out any time. I'll see you in a few hours."

"Thanks again so much for your help, Jim," said Jo. "I won't forget it."

She got out first and Morgan just grinned. Eli tapped him on the shoulder and said, "No funny ideas, Jim. She's spoken for."

Morgan looked at Eli with surprise. "Not you? Oh,

that's something new. I want to hear all about it on the way back to Miami."

"Don't hold your breath."

Morgan smiled again and said, "Two o'clock. Don't be late." The Suburban drove off down the parking area and Eli followed Jo up to lobby.

"You'll have to tell me about your friend Jim," she said as they walked back to their room. "He seems like a really nice guy."

Eli nodded. "Yes, he's great. A real prince." *If she only knew*, he thought.

Chapter 22

They sat silently together in the lobby, both lost in their own thoughts. Eli wondered if she'd agreed to that deal with Manuel, even though he was no longer able to fulfill his end. It weighed on his mind, as did her earlier comments about their relationship. He wanted to talk about it, to try and understand what her true feelings were, but it was neither the time nor the place. He didn't want to be confrontational, either. Eli realized he had that tendency, especially when his emotions were involved, but he vowed to hold back until they were safely in Miami and he could see her alone, with no outside distractions.

"What are you thinking about?" Eli asked.

"Lots of things. Mother and Father, the company, what I do now about pretty much everything."

He touched her hand and looked into her eyes.

"I'm really sorry about your parents. I'm sorry you had to find out this way, and I'm equally sorry they were involved in that whole mess."

She smiled and said, "I know. Thanks for that, but it's no one's fault but theirs. Mother just told me to mind my own business when I challenged her on her habit, said she could handle it and it was no big deal. And Father wouldn't listen when I tried to suggest ways to improve our product line. He was pretty stubborn about things in general, but when it came to McHenry-Taylor, he felt he was never wrong. I guess that's why he was so desperate in the end." She paused and sighed. "If it's anyone's fault it's really mine. I just couldn't get either one of them to budge."

"Jo, you did what you could. They were adults, after all, and capable of making their own decisions. You couldn't *make* them do the right things if they didn't want to. You can't blame yourself."

"Don't worry, Eli. I see the world in a pretty simple way. I know I'm not to blame, but I still feel sad. For now I'll focus on getting their affairs in order and filing for their death certificates. Maybe Leslie will have found something by now that will simplify things for me."

"Maybe. I'll call him as soon as we get back and see if he recovered anything from Joulters. I'll do whatever I can to help." He touched her hand again and she held it tightly.

"I know you will. Next up will be preparing for the Board meeting next week. I could really use some time to get my head straight after all this, but I'm afraid Lloyd will push the meeting forward with or without me. I have to have all my arguments ready and well thought out before that meeting." She paused for a second and added, "So how does it feel to be a millionaire?"

Eli hadn't stopped to consider that fact since she'd

handed him the check a week ago. He was momentarily dumbstruck by the thought. So much had happened since then, it seemed more like a dream than reality.

"I haven't really given it much thought," he replied. "I've been a little preoccupied until now. I guess it will hit me when we're back in Miami. You know, you way overpaid for what you got."

She smiled and her bright blue eyes flashed the way he remembered when he first met her.

"I think it was a bargain at twice the price."

"Oh, so maybe I should charge you another million?" mused Eli.

She laughed and pushed him away. "I don't think so. Besides, you got plenty of "fringe" benefits along the way."

Eli chuckled and shook his head. "Ok then, it's agreed. We have a fair deal. Shake?"

They shook hands and she kissed him on the cheek.

At that moment the bellman walked up and said, "Mr. Rose, yuh car is here." They followed him out with their small tote bags and he put them in the back of the Suburban.

"I hope yuh enjoyed yuh stay wit us. Please come back soon." He waved as they drove off down the hill.

Morgan spent much of the next hour regaling Jo with partially true stories of Eli's exploits, making sure to leave out the seamy details and negative aspects where appropriate. They arrived at the private plane gate and were admitted by the guard without question. The Suburban pulled up to a non-descript hanger and Morgan said, "Ok, we're here. Our ride is inside. Follow me."

He led the way into the building, which housed a new, dark gray unmarked Beechcraft Super King Air B300C, a Macchi AL 60-B2, and a Citation V Model 560. Eli knew that the "Beech" was standard DEA equipment, used for mostly for surveillance, but the Macchi was a plane he recognized from his days with The Agency. They often used them in Central America for short-range intelligence gathering missions, and he was surprised to see one there.

The engines on the Citation were already running and the walkway was down, awaiting their arrival. As they walked toward the unmarked plane, Eli said to Morgan, " I see you're peacefully co-exiting with the DEA."

Morgan looked back at him and yelled through the whine of the engines, "For now. We just recently got permission to use their hanger from time to time. We "borrowed" this baby from the Marines." He waved for Jo to climb up first and then waited for Eli, who followed her in.

Morgan had a quick word with one of the ground crew and then boarded. The co-pilot closed the door and returned to the cabin as the pilot began to taxi out of the hanger. The pilot came on the intercom and said, "All passengers please fasten your seatbelts and remain seated until further notice. Tower, this is Citation N407B requesting permission to depart. Roger, tower. Will taxi 10/28 and hold."

The engines whined loudly behind them as they approached the end of the runway. An ALM 737 came roaring down and made a perfect landing ahead of them and quickly cleared to the taxiway.

"Roger, tower. Citation N407B rolling," said the pilot. The co-pilot then closed the cabin door and the jet accelerated down the runway with a roar. The takeoff distance was very short compared to the civilian jets, and they were soon climbing to their cruising altitude en route to Miami.

Eli looked out the window as the island slipped out of sight, laid his head back in the seat and took a deep breath, feeling relieved again that they'd escaped without injury. He thought that if he ever returned he would try and locate Cokee-eye Arthur and thank him again for his help and good sense. Or maybe he wouldn't? He decided to think about it for awhile after they got back to Miami. Jo was already asleep and he felt like a long nap would be a great idea, too.

"Eli, now that Jo is out, I wanna' bring you up to speed on what's goin' on with this whole thing."

Eli groaned, realizing his nap might be postponed indefinitely. Morgan leaned in closer and said, "Vicente's been very busy while you've been out playin' games with your lady friend. Seems like he found out a few things about her family that aren't kosher."

"Spare me the details," said Eli wearily. "I already know about her parents."

Morgan nodded. "Ok, we'll skip that part. It turns out that he had to get cozy with Paco Gutiérrez to get the info, but he also had to demonstrate his value in the process. He's arranged for this sub of yours to offload its cargo in Pinar del Rio, then have the goods shipped to a small port in Yucatán where the Gulf Cartel will take possession of it. He made me promise to tip the

Coast Guard in your name so I placed a call to DOD and had them tell the Coast Guard that the tip came from you. The "Coasties" agreed to let the Colombians drop the cargo first before they try and nab them when they leave Cuban territorial waters."

"Very interesting. I'll have to have a talk with Vicente when I get back about minimizing his involvement in this type of stuff." Eli laid his head back against the seat again, but Morgan continued with his debriefing.

"That's the pot callin' the kettle black if I've ever heard it," laughed Morgan. "You're one to talk, with all the shit you get involved in."

"Give one example where I've crossed the line - recently," said Eli indignantly.

"Like how about right now. I'm havin' to bail you and your "hottie" out of a helluva' mess here. And don't think I don't know about what happened to Manuel Durán and his men. You really screwed that one up but good." Morgan grinned at him.

"Look, that wasn't me."

Morgan stared hard at Eli until he finally said, "Ok, fair enough. I promise I won't say anything to Vicente."

Morgan flashed a satisfied smile. "So, as I was sayin', Vicente got himself in pretty deep. Unfortunately, he didn't happen to know that a joint FBI-DEA-ATF task force called Orchid was watchin' Gutiérrez and preparin' a case against him."

That got Eli's rapt attention, and he said, "Oh, shit. So how much trouble is he in?"

"What he told me is that he has a deal with the task force to flip Gutiérrez and his boys once the drug deal is done. What that also tells me is that Vicente is plannin' to be in Mexico when the deal goes down, probably on Friday. Pretty dangerous behavior if you ask me. I just thought you should know."

"Thanks," Eli said. "Yeah, I needed to know that. I guess I know where I'll be this weekend."

"I've already talked to the higher-up's about this and I've been told to back off, so you can't count on me for support." Morgan seemed distressed having to tell Eli that last bit of news.

"Don't worry about it," Eli replied. "At least this time I know you won't help before the fact, not like in Nicaragua."

"Shit!" yelled Morgan, who then forced himself to whisper so as not to wake up Jo. "You know I had to do that. We never woulda' nailed Jasper if I hadn't let the Sandinistas grab you. I thought you woulda' gotten over that by now."

"Yeah, well my feet are still sore. You have no idea how bad that was."

"Ok, I admit we coulda' done it a different way, but it was all I had at the time. Cut me some slack here. I'm tryin' to make it up to you." Morgan seemed sincere, but Eli never knew if he really meant it when he sounded this way or it was just another act.

"Forget it," said Eli.

Morgan sat back and let a few seconds go by in silence. "I've got a job for your, Eli."

Eli looked at him with surprise. "Are you kidding me? What did we just talk about?"

"I know all that, but I said I'm tryin' to make it up to you. Besides, it's a simple job, a piece of cake."

"I've heard that before. If it's so simple, why don't you get one of your green field agents to handle it? Sounds like a good training exercise to me."

Morgan looked up and said, "You know what? That's a great idea. We can make it a trainin' exercise. Let me brief you on what we need to do. You see there's this "situation" we need to clean up in Venezuela, and............."

"No way!" said Eli forcefully.

"But I haven't even told you what it's all about."

"I don't care, I'm not doing it."

"But....."

"No. I'm not doing it. Find someone else."

Morgan sighed. "We can discuss it later, after you've had some time to relax and decompress from this one."

Eli looked into his eyes and said, "What is it about the word "no" that you don't understand?"

"Ok, Ok. I'll stop."

Morgan sat back in his seat and stared silently at the cabin door while Eli reclined his seat and quickly went to sleep. *I've got him back*, thought Morgan. *Finally, I've got him back.*

§

"Eli, wake up," said Jo. "We're almost there."

He stretched and looked out the window. They were flying over the Great Bahama Bank and were only a few minutes east of Miami.

"Thanks," he said. "Sorry I went out like that."

"Don't apologize. It's been a rough few days and we

both needed the sleep. You want to wake up your friend Jim?"

Eli looked over at Morgan, who had fallen asleep with his mouth wide open. He tapped him on the should and said, "Hey Jim. Jim, wake up. We'll be landing in a few minutes."

Morgan's eyes popped open and he quickly straightened himself up, brushing his few remaining strands of hair off his forehead with his hand.

The pilot came on the intercom again and said, "Will all passengers please be seated. Fasten your seatbelts and bring your seat backs to their full upright position. We will be on the ground shortly."

The late afternoon sun shone brightly through the left side windows so Morgan pulled them closed. The Citation bumped and rocked in the afternoon turbulence, dodging the numerous isolated thunderstorms that peppered their approach.

Eli looked down as they crossed over Miami Beach and wondered how Vicente and Rita were doing, now that they knew he was Ok. *She'll probably ignore me and pretend that it was no big deal*, he thought about Rita. But he knew differently.

They glided in smoothly with some last second adjustments just before they touched down, and then taxied over to a separate hanger away from the main terminals. Eli could see several DEA planes parked in front of the building and was glad that they would not have to clear customs and immigration with the hoard of travelers that usually choke that facility in the main building. *Morgan will have everything arranged. Good guy.*

The plane taxied into the hanger where the ground crew signaled them in and waved them clear. The pilot cut the engines and opened the cabin door, then the co-pilot stuck his head out and said, "Can I please have your passports? I will give them back to you in a few minutes. Please remain on the plane until the captain or I say you can leave."

He collected the documents and lowered the gangway, then went down the stairs to meet the waiting customs agent. Morgan watched to make sure there were no issues, and the agent quickly handed the passports back to the co-pilot. He climbed halfway up the stairs and said, "Alright. We're cleared for entry. Welcome back to the US."

Eli, Morgan, and Jo collected themselves and their small bags and thanked the captain as they left. Eli noted two black Ford Crown Victoria's waiting for them outside the hanger with their doors open and the motors running. They walked to the nearest one and Morgan said, "Well Miss McHenry. It's been a real pleasure meetin' you. I hope the rest of your issues can be worked out without too much trouble."

Jo reached over and kissed him on the cheek. "Thank you so much for your help. You're a real life saver. I hope one day I can repay the favor." She hugged him and turned to Eli.

"I don't really know what else to say that I haven't already told you. Thank you for finding out what happened to my parents, and for bringing me peace. I'll call you this weekend." She pressed herself against him as hard as someone could and hugged him for several seconds. Then she got into the car and drove off.

Eli felt empty and weak but focused on what he still needed to do before the day was over.

"Jim, I need to go to the office. Vicente and Rita will be.........."

"I had my people here contact them and send them home. We told them you were Ok and would be back in the office tomorrow morning." Eli started to protest but Morgan continued. "You can make whatever arrangements with Vicente you need to make over the phone tonight or in the office tomorrow. Right now, it is my opinion, as your former senior officer, that you need some rest in your own bed. We're gonna' drop you at your place. No arguments, that's where this car is headed. Got it?"

"Got it," Eli answered, shaking his head.

They rode back to his condo building on Brickell Avenue and Eli just stared out at the traffic the entire trip. Before he realized where they were they had pulled up outside his building, the Villa Regina. He'd picked up his two bedroom place for a great price only a few months before, and it was extremely convenient to the office, a reasonably short walk or a two minute drive if the weather was bad.

"Thanks for the ride, Morgan. I guess we'll be in touch."

"No problem, Eli. I consider us even now. I'll be expectin' to hear from you when this shit with the Colombians is all cleaned up."

They shook hands and Eli just nodded.

"Don't go gettin' yourself killed. And keep Vicente outta' trouble while you're at it." Morgan smiled and patted him on the back. Eli got out and went into the building, then rode the elevator up to his place. He threw his bag on the sofa and called Vicente at home.

"Vicente, Jo and I are back. Just wanted to let you know I'll be in tomorrow and we can work out whatever is still hanging over your head with your other issue."

"Eli, thanks to God you are back safe. I worry so much. You are Ok? How is Jo?"

"She's doing well, all things considered. She's got a lot of things to handle in the next few days, so I don't expect we'll hear from her for awhile."

"*Si*, I understand. Ok, you get some rest now and we talk in the morning. There is time to do whatever is necessary. Good night my friend."

"See you tomorrow."

Eli hung up and wandered over to his refrigerator with the intent to eat something. He was hungry but didn't have the energy to get cleaned up enough to go out, even though he suspected his food had spoiled by now. He smelled the milk and it had definitely soured, and he guessed the cold cuts he'd bought the previous week were probably past their prime as well. So he got a glass of water and had a few sips, then collapsed on the sofa and turned on the television to watch the Channel 6 news.

He tuned in just in time to hear the commentator say, "In international news today, the government of Trinidad and Tobago made public a reported shoot out between rival drug cartels in the eastern part of the country. An unknown number of people are said to have died in the violence, which also involved the burning of a major structure. So far the police have no leads and are still investigating. In China today, the........."

Eli turned it off. So that was as much of an epitaph as Manuel would ever know. A footnote on the evening news, and he wasn't even mentioned by name. *What a stupid waste*, he thought. He laid his head back against the cushion and almost instantly fell asleep.

He awoke to the phone ringing, and stumbled over to answer it. The sun was shining in his balcony door and he looked at his watch. *Nine o'clock. Holy shit*! He guessed it would be Rita on the line, making sure he was up and Ok.

"Eli, what the hell is going on?" she said.

"What do you mean?"

"You get in after all that, all that worry and you can't even call me? You are an SOB, you know that?" She was really mad, but Eli knew it wouldn't last.

"I'm sorry, Ok? I called Vicente last night and told him I'd be in this morning."

"Great. So where the hell are you?"

"I overslept."

"Well get in here as soon as you can. There's a lot of shit going on and Vicente is getting nervous again." She didn't even wait for him to acknowledge that last comment before she hung up.

Great. Welcome back, he thought. Eli dragged himself to the shower and doused himself in the hot water for fifteen minutes. He finally felt clean and the shower energized him. He threw on a pair of buff-colored Ralph Lauren trousers and a pressed white shirt and went down to the garage. The GTO started right up and that made him happy, so he drove the short hop over to the office.

When he walked into the office Rita was waiting for him with a big cup of *café cubano* and the sports section from the *Herald.* She gave him a big hug and pressed herself against him in a more than friendly way.

"Hi boss. It's good to have you back."

He smiled and patted her round rear. "It's good to be back."

"Hey, watch the harassment!" she said, smiling.

Eli put the paper on his desk and took the coffee with him to see Vicente.

"Hey, old man, how are you doing?"

Vicente immediately jumped up and hugged his former *protégé.* "Is so good to see you, Eli. I so happy you are Ok."

"Good to see you, too. So," he said, sitting down to sip his coffee, "tell me about all this mess with Paco Gutiérrez. What have you gotten yourself into now?"

Vicente recounted how he'd worked through Enrique Ramírez to find out about the McHenrys financial and other affairs, and contacted Julio Villareal for help setting up the Cuba drop for Paco Gutiérrez. He told him again about his meeting with Lloyd Taylor, his meetings with Paco and the FBI, and the details of the plans to move the drugs.

"You have been a busy guy, Vicente," said Eli. "So how is the Orchid task force going to close this out?"

"I do not know. This guy Rodríguez, he no contact me yet."

"Well, then it's time we contact him. We need to

know how long we'll have to stay with Gutiérrez in case we have to plan our own escape, if it comes to that."

Vicente was concerned and it showed on his haggard face.

"Eli, you no can be involve. Paco, he a very suspicious guy. If I bring a new person to the meetings maybe he has too much worry and call off the drop."

Eli seriously considered Vicente's concerns. "There is that risk, but based on what you told me about the operation, I think he has no other option but to go through with the deal. You see, his boss, the guy that handles distribution in the Caribbean, was "offed" by the Jamaicans a couple of days ago, so Paco can't send the stuff back where it came from. It's either Cuba or dump it in the ocean, and I'm betting he wants his cut too much to sacrifice it. He'll go through with the plan, you can believe it."

"I hope you are right," said Vicente, rubbing his forehead nervously.

Eli heard the phone ring at Rita's desk and she appeared in the doorway looking worried.

"Vicente, there's a guy on the phone. He sounds like a *Colombiano* and he's asking for you."

"Thank you, Rita. Please, you can connect him." Vicente looked up at Eli and raised his eyebrows. "So you see, now it begin." He picked up the receiver and said in Spanish, "Vicente Amarón speaking. Who calls?"

Eli couldn't make out the voice on the other end of the line, but Vicente's expression looked pained. "*Si, si.* I understand. We can be there in one hour. *Si,* of course.

Ok, see you soon."

He put down the phone and with a deep sigh, sat back in his chair. "We must call Rodríguez now," he said. "That was one of Paco's guys. He wants me to come to his place in one hour. I think maybe he want to keep me close until the deal is done. Rodríguez must know."

"I guess there's no choice," said Eli. "Tell him we'll meet him at the park in ten minutes. We need to get over to Paco's place on time, especially because you're going to introduce your "partner" to him. We can take your car because it has that RFID device on it, and if anything happens, at least we'll know where to find it later." He got up while Vicente called Rodríguez and went in to talk to Rita.

"Rita, honey, I need you to listen and not ask questions. Vicente and I are going to be gone for a few days. I want you to leave the office about thirty minutes after us and go visit your sister in Orlando until Monday. Understand?

"Eli, Vicente told me the same thing. What's going on?" she said, clearly concerned.

"I'm not going to lie to you. We're likely going to be "required" to stay with this guy Gutiérrez until the transfer is completed in Mexico and the FBI and DEA have busted him. It could get real nasty and I don't want you hanging around, just in case someone comes looking for us. You got it?" He stared hard at her, and she realized he meant business, and there was no point in protesting.

"I got it," said Rita, downcast. Vicente came out and nodded at Eli, and Rita grabbed his arm as he turned to leave. "Guys, please be careful. I don't know what I'd do if........."

"You just do what I said," repeated Eli. "Don't worry about us. You know we're a good team."

Eli smiled and Vicente waved at her and they were gone. Rita began to tear up but forced herself to concentrate of shutting down the office. The minutes passed agonizingly slowly, but she obediently stayed in the office until exactly thirty minutes had passed, then locked the door and went down to the garage, not knowing if she'd ever see her guys again.

She felt bad about leaving, abandoning them when they needed her the most. *I can't just leave them out there with no support. What if they need me and I'm not there?* She wrestled with her feelings and with the instructions Eli had just given her, knowing that he wouldn't have told her to go if he hadn't had a good reason. She stopped with her key in the car door.

I just can't do this to them, she decided. *I'll stay, just in case.* Regardless of what Eli had told her, she would be there by the telephone until they returned. *That's my job and that's what I'm going to do, no matter what.*

Chapter 23

"So where is he?" said Eli, nervously glancing at his watch. "We can't be late to Paco's."

"There," said Vicente. "There he is."

Rodríguez was walking quickly to avoid breaking into a run. He paused for a second as he approached when he realized that Vicente was not alone.

"Ok, Vicente, What's so important you had to pull me out of a logistics meeting? And who's this?"

"Thank you for meet with us. This is Eli Rose. He was work the connection from another angle and he is here to help. Listen because we no have much time. Paco want me to come to his place right now. I think he will keep us until the exchange in Mexico on Friday. I will no have contact with you, so you have to move quickly."

Rodríguez said, "Shit! Ok, we can deal with it. I have to set things in motion with the Mexican PJF but we can be there as planned. What time is the handover?"

"If it go Ok, maybe two or three in the afternoon."

The agent looked at his watch and said, "I'll tell

Smith. You guys do what you need to do. If there is any change in plans you've got to find a way to get a message out to me. Otherwise, the next time we meet will be when we take these assholes down."

"Ok," said Vicente. "We understand. *Vaya con Dios, amigo.*"

"And you too, go with God. Good luck."

Rodríguez ran back towards the task force office while Vicente and Eli walked quickly to the Corvette and drove off.

They arrived at the massive, wrought iron gates of Paco's house with five minutes to spare and pushed the buzzer.

"Who is?" said the highly accented voice in English.

"Vicente, with someone."

The was a pause and then the gate opened. Vicente drove in and parked behind the black Mercedes. The two men got out and pressed the buzzer at the door, and were let in by one of the bodyguards.

"Vicente, down here," said Paco in English, waving from a corner of the sunken living room. As was his style, he sat on a large sofa in the midst of five beautiful young girls who were clad in very short skirts and skimpy tops. The man himself wore a white linen shirt, open to the waist with matching trousers.

"So, I see you brought a guest? Who is this?"

"Eli Rose," said Eli, presenting himself. He offered his hand but Paco did not move to shake it. "I am Vicente's partner."

Paco looked at Vicente and smiled.

"Girls, run off and find something fun to do. I need to have a talk with these gentlemen." The girls all got up and filed out onto the patio. When they had left, Paco's expression turned cold and menacing.

"Vicente, *amigo,* what are you thinking?" he said, putting his arm around the older man's shoulder. "You come to my house with some dick that I don't know and expect me to just accept him, like nothing is wrong? What the hell are you thinking?" He grabbed Vicente by the back of the neck and squeezed.

To his credit, Vicente stayed calm and played the submissive role he'd assumed on his earlier visits.

"Look, I no try and mess things up. Eli, he is my partner. He must be involve at some point. We are get close now so I think that maybe is time for you two to meet."

Paco turned to face Eli and stood very close to him. "You never told me you had a partner. I don't like that idea so much. Maybe I don't like any of this. Maybe I should have Rudy here put a bullet in your ear and dump you in the bay."

Eli stared at Paco, who stared back at him without blinking.

"Paco," Vicente stammered, "is really no problem. You no want Eli involve, is Ok. What you think, Eli?"

Eli stared hard at Paco and said, "Whatever you want, Vicente. You want me to leave, I'll leave."

Paco smiled and stepped back towards Vicente, putting his arm around his shoulder again.

"You know what, Vicente? Maybe it's a good idea to have another guy along, just to make sure everything works out the way it's supposed to. The more, the merrier, like the *gringo's* say. And I can keep my eye on you two and make sure you don't try to pull anything."

He laughed and Vicente forced himself to laugh as well. Eli allowed himself a thin smile but continued to stare at Paco.

"So, everything's cool, right? Good. Let me tell why I called you here. You boys are coming with me to Mexico to oversee the transfer of the cargo. We're going to leave tomorrow night, after your guys start unloading the sub. I have a private charter that will fly us directly to Mérida. We will have two cars to take us to Chiquilá, and my contact tells me that Juan Garcia-Puli himself is going to meet us there."

Eli recognized that name. He struggled for a second to remember where he'd heard it but then grasped what Paco meant.

"He's the head of the Gulf Cartel, isn't he?"

"Very good, Eli. You know your stuff. Yeah, he's the big deal in Mexico right now, so a visit from him is no small thing." Paco sat back down on the sofa with his arms outstretched.

"Pretty soon, you guys are going to be living the good life like me. We have twenty tons of blow to deliver, enough to keep all the rich *gringo's* high for at least a week, once it's cut."

"Paco, I must be able to make a phone call on Thursday night to confirm the exchange. You no have a problem with this?" Vicente played the part of a timid crook very well. He almost had Eli convinced he'd lost his nerve.

"No. No problem, as long as we can listen in."

Vicente nodded and Paco smiled.

"Ok, boys. Since we're going to be roommates for awhile, we might as well have some fun. Hey, Rudy. Call the girls back in. I want them to meet our new friend Eli."

Rudy leaned out onto the patio and called for the girls to come back to the house. They pranced in and sat around Paco like he was their benefactor.

"Ladies, this is Eli. He's Vicente's partner. Make him feel at home." Paco smiled and put his arm around the girl that sat on his right. Two young, buxom girls with long black hair approached Eli and stood on either side of him.

"Go on Eli. The girls will show you a good time."

"No doubt," Eli said, eyeing the girls. "But I don't mix business with pleasure, so I'll take a rain check until after our trip, if that's Ok with you."

Paco smiled and shook his head. "Whatever you want. So make yourself at home. Hey Rudy - call Juan Francisco and get him over here right away. I can't show up for a meeting with the *Mexicanos* with these two looking like this."

Eli and Vicente looked at each other quizzically. Before either could respond, Paco added, "Let's get them in some decent clothes, Armani or something. Tell Juan to bring everything they'll need." Rudy nodded and ran off to make his call, leaving Eli and Vicente perplexed.

"You guys will have to spend some of your green on some decent clothes if you're going to hang with me." Paco seemed satisfied with his control of the situation, so he turned his attention back to the girls that draped themselves on him like happy kittens.

Eli and Vicente sat down at the dining room table and waited for Paco's personal tailor, Juan Francisco to arrive. Eli wondered if he'd be like his father, a serious craftsman with years of experience or a young guy like Paco, short on experience but big on ideas. An hour later he saw that Juan Francisco was the former, a small, thin man older than Vicente, sporting a large gray mustache and a haggard looking face.

The old tailor immediately greeted Paco with a bow and waved for his helpers to bring in the clothes from his van.

"Juan, I want you to make these two guys look presentable, you know, like the rest of the boys." Paco waved at his other bodyguards, who were in the den playing cards.

"*Si Señor* Gutiérrez," said Juan Francisco with a slight bow. He turned his attention to Vicente first and reached for a light gray silk Armani suit jacket. "You try," he said in heavily accented English.

Vicente greeted him in Spanish and Juan Francisco smiled for the first time. He helped Vicente into the jacket and smoothed the shoulders. He made two chalk marks at the sleeves and waist and then asked Vicente to try on the trousers. Vicente looked at Rudy, who motioned for him to follow him to the bathroom. Juan Francisco then turned his attention to Eli and handed him a charcoal gray Armani jacket. He fussed with the sleeves and taper for a second and then waved for Eli to try on the trousers as well.

When they had completed their fittings, the old tailor mixed and matched several shirts and ties with each suit to be sure of the combinations.

"Ok, I bring back in two hours," he said hoarsely. Before he left, he handed three shirts to each man, plus socks, underwear, and the ties. Then he left with his assistant, bowing slightly to Paco before exiting the front door.

"He's a real trip," said Paco. "He'll have you fixed up in no time."

"Thank you," said Vicente. "This is a very nice thing you do."

"Got to present the right image. Can't have you two looking like department store goons when we meet Garcia-Puli. We got to look the part."

Eli smiled and nodded and gave no outward sign of his disgust with the young guy. He held his clothes and walked over to the den to watch the card game, which had become animated and fairly loud since Juan Francisco's departure. Vicente joined him, and they each found a comfortable chair to sit and watch the action.

Over the years, Eli and Vicente's long association and close relationship helped them form a familial bond, and that was clear to all who knew them away from the office. However, it also contributed to their almost uncanny ability to read each other's facial expressions and anticipate each other's actions. After an hour of watching Paco's men joke and curse each other as they played cards, Eli and Vicente had become part of the game, mixing in like old friends and sharing the barbs like they'd known the others for years. Eli knew that this was a good way to assess their personalities;

which one was a hot-head, which one was conservative, which one a risk-taker and which one shunned risks. It was a critical element in his planning for when they would need to separate themselves from the group in Mexico.

Vicente seemed to understand as well, and played into the verbal jousting by reminding Alvaro and Rudy of their first meeting. They didn't smile until their mates piled on, ribbing Rudy about the condition of his "package" after Vicente's well-placed kick. Alvaro suffered as well, hearing from the crowd about how Vicente had improved his looks by re-arranging his nose. Everyone laughed, and Eli shot a quick glance at Vicente, who winked in reply.

They continued to get close to their new compatriots throughout the day. Rudy confided to Eli that each of the men had been fitted for a wardrobe by the old tailor for the same reason that he and Vicente had been fitted: Paco wanted all his guys to look the part as well as play the part of tough drug dealers.

"He think maybe this is *Miami Vice*," said Rudy in a whisper. But he was happy to get the clothes, as were the others, since they had come off the street with next to nothing. Even though they thought of Paco as a preening poseur, they still appreciated his generosity and were fiercely loyal.

He's managed to do something right, Eli thought. Loyalty in this situation was hard to measure and even harder to count on, but he believed that Paco knew what it took to earn it from his men. He would not underestimate any of them in a fight, especially if Paco was threatened in any way.

Juan Francisco returned late in the afternoon with their suits and a pair of black Bruno Magli wingtip shoes and matching Moreschi belts for each of them. He smiled weakly at Vicente and then approached Paco, speaking in hushed tones that Eli could not make out. The old tailor nodded and bowed again, then left as before without speaking.

Eli went to the bathroom and changed clothes, marveling at the fit. *I need to find this guy when this is over*, he thought. Even the shoes were comfortable and fit without pinching or slipping. Vicente then changed and afterwards they went back to the den to watch a tape of the movie *Scarface* with their newfound friends. The guards were hooting with laughter at the caricature of ruthless Cuban drug dealer Tony Montana.

"Look at this shit!" yelled Alvaro. "Nobody would ever follow this guy, the way he treats people," he added, looking at Eli.

Eli nodded and smiled. They laughed and yelled at the screen every time Tony Montana made a crack about the drug business or how he would deal with his rivals. They mocked the characters and the story, yet seemed to be living the story, or at least part of it. They oscillated between mimicking and mocking entertainment like *Miami Vice* or *Scarface*, poking fun when it was uncomfortable or outrageous, yet emulating many of the attitudes and behaviors espoused by the main characters. Eli found it hypocritical, yet surprisingly consistent. He leaned over to Vicente and said, "Wake me up if something happens."

Vicente nodded and Eli took off his new jacket and hung it on the back of one of the dining room chairs, then fell sound sleep amid the raucous outbursts of his new "team."

The entire household was tense by Thursday afternoon. Paco had banished the girls to the patio once again, tiring of their feigned affection and idle chatter. The guards alternately wandered the grounds or nervously cleaned their weapons, unclear about whether or not they'd need them. Eli and Vicente took turns speaking with each man privately, again trying to glean some understanding of their characters and motivations. They felt like they understood the others pretty well by the evening, well enough to relax before Vicente's call to Julio.

At ten o'clock, Vicente asked for the telephone and with Paco listening on another line, called Julio at his new camp in Perrine. That's where he kept the radio he used to communicate with his network in Cuba, and he answered as planned.

"Who calls?"

"Vicente is calling. What is the status of the operation?"

"Let me make the call. I will have some news in ten minutes."

"Ok," said Vicente, and Julio hung up.

Paco conveyed a puzzled look from across the room but Vicente just smiled and waved. He called again after the ten minutes had elapsed and this time Julio had something to tell him.

"The transfer is taking place now. There was a problem in the beginning but it goes Ok now."

"What kind of problem?" asked Vicente.

"The captain does not speak Spanish, only English and Russian. We were not able to communicate for the first twenty minutes. We have everything under control now. The work will be done in another thirty minutes. The other ship is standing by off the coast. We have been speaking with him and he will come in as soon as the Russians leave."

Paco looked over at Vicente and shrugged, not clearly understanding what was taking place.

"Ok, very good," answered Vicente. "I will call you in the usual place on Monday."

Julio hung up without another word. Paco handed the telephone to Rudy and walked over to Vicente.

"So, what's going on? Are we ready to go or what?"

"That depends."

"Depends on what?" Paco replied, a bit agitated.

"If you trust that the other boat is loaded Ok, we can go now to Mexico. The boat should arrive between two and three tomorrow afternoon. If you want confirmation of the time, it will be more than one hour and a half more."

Paco looked at his huge gold Rolex and shook his head.

"No, I think we can do this. Rudy - call the plane. Tell them we'll be at the airport in an hour. Pick your best five guys and let's go." He looked at Vicente and Eli and said, "You guys ride with me."

The black Mercedes and one of the Suburbans were parked outside with their doors open and the motors running when Paco, Eli, and Vicente came out. Rudy rode with his team in the Suburban so Eli sat in the front of the Mercedes with the driver. They sped off and were buzzed quickly through the gate. Vicente thought of Special Agent Rodríguez as they drove and hoped he'd have a team in place as planned. There was no way to signal him to let him know where they were leaving from and when they were going, so it he hoped he'd be in Chiquilá at the right time.

For his part, Eli hoped that the Coast Guard was able to intercept the submarine, and he thought about Jo and wondered how she was and if she was ready for the Board meeting.

Paco noted his companions silence and bumped Vicente on the shoulder.

"Come on, guys. Why you looking so nervous? Got something to worry about that I should know?"

Vicente smiled at Paco and shook his head.

"No, Paco. I think about my friends in Pinar. I hope he is Ok. Is very hard for me not to know. Maybe I can call at the airport?"

"Don't worry, buddy. You sound more like an old woman than an old man. Everything is fine; you told me yourself. Nothing can go wrong, eh *amigo*?"

Eli continued to stare straight ahead, doing his best to ignore Paco.

"And you? What's on your mind, Eli?"

Eli sighed and looked back at Paco. Before he could answer, Vicente cut in and said, "He think about a lady."

Paco smiled. "Is that so? You thinking about a chick, Eli? She must really be something?"

"Yep, she's one of a kind," Eli replied.

Paco slapped Eli on the forearm in a friendly gesture of kinship.

"Well, don't worry about her. If she takes off you can have one of mine. That girl Lucy, let me tell you, she will screw your brains out. She'll make you forget that other girl, trust me. And if she ain't good enough, I'll get you a better one. If this goes as planned, the sky's the limit *amigo*. Anything you want, just ask and it's yours."

"Very generous," said Eli smiling weakly. He decided to change the subject while there was a break in Paco's train of thought.

"By the way, where are we flying out of?"

"Tamiami," said Paco. "I have a Citation III ready to go. We get on, take off, no questions asked. Simple as it can be."

"Simple," Eli repeated. Paco smiled and sat back in his seat, staring out the window as the caravan sped his towards southwest Miami.

They arrived at the private hanger after eleven thirty and found the jet ready to go with its engines already running. The Mercedes pulled up beside the Citation and Paco led the way to the stairs. Vicente paused for a second to see if there was a telephone within reach but thought the better of it and continued on. Eli, Rudy, and the rest of the team formed a line and followed them onto the plane.

Eli sat back and fastened his seat belt. He was ready to be done with Paco and his "boys" but had to tough it out one more time, he hoped. The plane taxied out a short distance and was on the runway in a few seconds. The pilot revved the engines and they roared to life, pressing the passengers back into their seats with perceptible force.

Eli looked over as the plane banked west and could see most of suburban Miami stretched out below. Millions of twinkling lights contributed to the glow of the city, which reflected off the scattered low clouds in shades of purple and amber. Their steep rate of climb abruptly flattened out and they banked slightly southwest, quickly passing over the Keys and the open ocean below.

"Attention, this is the captain speaking." The intercom was painfully loud.

"Our flight time to Mérida, Mexico will be approximately one and a half hours. You are free to move around the cabin until we are on final approach."

Vicente sat next to Paco, who was talking and gesticulating dramatically about something. He smiled and patted Vicente on the shoulder frequently, which signaled that everything was going well. At least Eli didn't have to listen to the little shit for the whole flight.

Eli laid his head back and looked out at the inky black ocean. The full moon finally broke through the scattered clouds along the coast and shone brightly, illuminating the water directly below them. It was strangely relaxing, almost hypnotic, and Eli dozed off, still thinking of Jo.

Chapter 24

He was jolted awake by the sudden bump. It lifted Eli out of his seat and the shouts that accompanied the disturbance shocked his senses. He looked around to find his traveling companions buckled in and gripping their armrests tightly.

"This is the captain. Nothing to worry about there, folks. Just some clear air turbulence as we approach the coast. Probably best for everyone to remain seated with your seatbelts fastened for the remainder of the flight. We should be on the ground in fifteen minutes."

The plane steadied and Eli sat back in his seat and relaxed again. They descended smoothly towards the airport and finally he could see the lights of Mérida as they passed overhead. The city was brightly lit but Eli couldn't see much from his side of the aircraft until the captain banked to the left. The view revealed the large downtown area with its central square and large cathedral, the common plan for almost every city and town in Latin America.

Eli could see the north-south runway as the captain aligned the plane and they descended rapidly to a soft landing. They taxied off quickly towards the private hangers and parked the jet next to another Citation, just in front of the buildings. Two white Chevy Suburbans sat just beside the administration buildings waiting for the newly arrived passengers. Rudy exited first along with the rest of his team, and they walked over to meet the drivers and get the vehicles ready for the others.

Paco stood near the exit and watched Rudy until he waved, indicating it was Ok to approach the vehicles. The air conditioners were running full blast when Paco, Eli, and Vicente climbed into the second Suburban. The Mexican driver greeted Paco and explained they would take him to a guest house just near the airport so they could all catch a few hours of sleep before their long drive. Paco just waved at the guy and they fell in behind the first vehicle, driving out to the main security gate. The guard approached the driver's side of Rudy's Suburban and stuck his head in the window for a moment, then emerged quickly and waved both vehicles through the gate.

The two Suburbans drove south along the airport boundary road for a few minutes and then turned west, passing through run-down neighborhoods with alternating stretches of paved and dirt roads. The streetlights dimly lit their way, illuminating only the area just below the lights. Initially they could see that most of the homes were of poor circumstances, but they soon arrived in a better neighborhood where the homes were newer and larger. They parked next to a tree-covered walkway and the driver indicated that they had reached their destination, a set of four new stucco and red-tiled bungalows that bordered a large swimming pool.

Paco got out and waited for Rudy to provide some signal that all was well. Two of the other guards ran into the first bungalow and soon returned, smiling and talking loudly. Rudy waved again and Eli and Vicente followed Paco up the walkway and into the first bungalow.

"I am Felipe Borador, the owner of this place," said a short, fat guy as he approached Paco. He extended his hand and smiled.

"It is a pleasure to be of service, *Señor* Gutiérrez."

Paco shook his hand. "So all this belongs to you? Very nice."

"Yes. The vehicles you will travel in tomorrow are mine also. I have provided some food by the pool for your men, and there are some girls there if they want to relax."

"Excellent," said Paco. "You have thought of everything, and I am very grateful. Is there anything you want from me?"

The little guy thought for a second before he spoke. He seemed reticent to mention what was on his mind, but realized there was no better time to speak up then right now.

"Well, there is one thing. Can you please mention to *Señor* Garcia-Puli that I assisted you?"

"Sure, of course," replied Paco, patting the guy on the shoulder.

Borador wiped the sweat from his forehead with a white handkerchief and a smile. He bowed slightly to Paco and shouted to the girls in Spanish, "You be nice to these Cuban boys. No complaints, or you'll answer to me!" He smiled again and left them alone in the bungalow.

The rooms were sparse but clean. The floors were of red Saltillo tile and the walls were a light terra cotta stucco on the inside. Each bungalow had a bathroom and three small beds, plus a window air conditioner and a small black and white television. The towels and linens looked clean and there was a small bar of soap at each sink. *Perfectly acceptable*, thought Eli.

"Rudy!" yelled Paco. Rudy ran over and Paco put his arm over his shoulder.

"Listen, I want you to tell the guys that we will be leaving here at eight tomorrow morning. It's going to take us about four hours to get there, and we don't want to be late. They can do whatever they want but they better be rested and looking good when we leave. Understand?"

Rudy stared at his boss and nodded. "Yes, boss. No problem, I will be sure they are ready to go."

"Ok, then, you go have some fun with the boys. But not *too* much fun."

Rudy smiled and hurried off to join his team.

"Gentlemen, you'll excuse me but I'm going to try and get some sleep before we go. Don't miss the departure hour tomorrow. I'll be pretty pissed off if Rudy has to come and find you." Paco looked at Vicente expectantly so Vicente nodded.

"Good. I'm going to take that one over there. You two should plan on sharing one of the others. We can let the boys have this one and that one over there." He pointed to his right. "Good night, gentlemen."

"Good night, Paco," said Vicente.

He looked at Eli and motioned for them to go to the far bungalow. They walked off around the end of the pool, glancing over to watch their compatriots eating and cavorting with the whores provided by Borador.

"You can pick whichever bed you want," said Eli as they entered the far bungalow.

The beds all looked the same so Vicente picked one nearest the door and stripped down to his underwear. He neatly hung his suit in on the hangers provided in the small closet and headed for the bathroom.

"Eli, you want this first?" he said, motioning towards the shower.

"No, that's Ok. You go first."

Eli hung his suit up and stretched out on the hard bed, lost in thought. He closed his eyes for just a second but was awakened by Vicente, who tapped him on the arm.

"Is for you now," he said.

Eli showered and set the alarm on his watch for five fifteen. He looked over to say good night to Vicente, but he was already sound asleep. *Good idea*, he thought. *It will be a hell of a day tomorrow, so let's get as much rest as possible.*

§

The alarm startled him when it went off but did its job well. Eli sat up and turned on the lamp next to the bed.

"Vicente, wake up. Time to get ready."

Vicente groaned and rolled over, throwing his legs

off the bed as if they were dead weights.

"I too old for this," he muttered on his way to the bathroom.

"That make's two of us," added Eli.

They dressed and made their way back to the pool where a large breakfast had been laid out. Several of the guards were also there, drinking coffee and eating silently. The distractions of the previous evening had obviously taken their toll on the group, but they seemed ready for the long drive and business ahead of them.

Paco emerged from the other far bungalow looking sharp and fresh. Maybe it was a shot of strong coffee or the adrenaline rush of knowing what lay ahead, but he was smiling and energetic. He greeted each his "boys" and patted them on the shoulder, joking with them about their fling with the Mexican girls. Many responded with a weak smile, but they smiled nonetheless.

Eli and Vicente gulped the coffee and ate some fresh *lechoza* and mango, then left the pool area and stood by second Suburban.

"I see you guys are ready to go and get this thing done. Good, I like that." Paco wandered out with a cup of coffee and joined them at the vehicle.

"We'll do the deal before the end of the day and be back in Miami for a good night's sleep."

"Is great, Paco," said Vicente.

The others arrived with Rudy, who had rounded up the Mexican drivers and they got into the vehicles and drove off on the Periferico loop road towards Federal Highway 180. This was the only road that connected Mérida with Cancún and the Riviera Maya on the east coast, and was as close to a highway as there could be through the forests of northern Yucatán.

As was typical for a summer morning, clouds were building to the south over the rainforest and the traffic east was thick with all manner of trucks, hauling everything from food to carpets. A fair number of painfully lethargic busses dotted the highway ahead of them as well, dutifully carrying their loads of workers to the tourist hotels and restaurants in Cancún. The early busses had long departed, so these transported the individuals that would stay late to see that their tourist guests were well attended.

The white Suburbans weaved through the dense traffic in fits and starts, the Mexican drivers squeezing into spaces between the busses and trucks where there did not seem to be enough room to fit a bicycle. This continued for almost an hour until they reached the toll road interchange at the town of Kantunil. From there, Highway 180 splits into two separate roads: one stays to the north and becomes a toll road that leads directly to Cancún, while the other stops at all the small villages that cross the flat jungle, and eventually leads to the famous Mayan ruins at Chichen Itza.

Most of the busses turned off onto the *Carretera Libre*, or Free Road once they cleared the toll plaza. Some of the trucks and private vehicles continued on the northern spur, the *Carretera Cuota*, or Toll Road, and the Suburbans were able to make up some of the time they'd lost on the way from Mérida. The driver leaned back and told Paco that they would be at the turn for Chiquilá in a little less than two hours, and he should let him know if he wanted to stop for a break. The roads north were in much worse condition and the towns were much smaller, so the trip was about to become as uncomfortable as it was monotonous. Paco told the driver to push on, so they continued to follow the first vehicle without signaling for them to stop.

Vicente and Paco both dozed as the big SUV's sped east. Clouds continued to build over the central Yucatán and Eli hoped they could get to the coast before the big storms began to move in. Eli was again in the uncomfortable position of having to rely on someone else's plan for their escape and recovery, and he always hated being in that situation.

The last time that happened was with Morgan in Nicaragua, and that ended badly for him, so he was equally nervous about trusting his life to an agent he barely knew from some likely dysfunctional joint agency task force. But escaping into the jungles of Quintana Roo seemed pointless, since the cartels basically operated openly there and had allies in every town and village. Eli could never get himself and Vicente safely out of Mexico if they were running from the Gulf Cartel, he reasoned. His mood darkened, and he sat glumly next to the driver, who cheerily played *Son Yucateco* and *Danza* music incessantly on the radio while they sped east.

Eli had a headache, and the *Danza* beamed in from Cancún wasn't helping. The lead Suburban began to slow down and he noticed that they were about to turn. He shifted in his seat and the driver leaned over and said, "El Ideal. We go north here. Then we stop at Kantunil Kín. *Gasolina.*"

Eli only nodded. Their small caravan turned left and they were off on the two lane road north to Chiquilá.

They covered miles of rutted road, acceptable in places and pock marked in others, but needed only thirty minutes to reach the jungle town of Kantunil Kín. The drivers were very mindful of the speed limit signs along the way, as these roads were notorious for speed traps set up by the Mexican police. They were a good source of extra "fees" collected by the individual officers on behalf of the local municipalities, but usually pocketed by the officers in return for your passport or drivers license.

They passed slowly through the arched entrance gate and into the sleepy town. Paco woke up and stared silently out the window for a few seconds.

"Where the hell are we?" he said.

"Some place called Kantunil Kín," Eli answered. "The driver said they need gas, so I guess we'll have a pit stop. I don't think we have much farther to go."

Paco looked at his watch with some concern.

"Well, we better not waste any time here 'cause we're already running behind schedule." He tapped the driver on the shoulder and said in Spanish, "When we stop, you tell the other guy that we have to make up some time. I want to be in Chiquilá by one fifteen at the latest."

"Ok, *Señor* Gutiérrez. No problem."

The lead vehicle suddenly hit the brakes and turned in to a PEMEX gas station just down the road on the right. The two SUV's jammed in next to each other and Paco's driver yelled out instructions to his partner. The guy nodded and waved and shouted at the attendant, "Fill the tank with red, please." *Rojo*, or red as it is known is the premium fuel sold by the state oil company at its stations, and both vehicles were hooked up to the pumps immediately.

Paco, Eli and Vicente got out and wandered into the store where Vicente managed to wrangle the bathroom key from a disinterested young guy behind the counter. The group queued up and when each one was done, they bought soft drinks and snacks for the road. The drivers paid for the gas and the team piled back into the vehicles, refreshed and awake.

The road deteriorated as the Suburbans continued north, so their progress was slow and uncomfortable. They passed through the small villages of San Ángel and Solferino and Eli reminded himself of how futile any escape would be if they had to flee on foot. The further north they drove, the more swampy the area became. The place was filled with mosquitoes and poisonous snakes, and away from the villages and only road lay misery and certain death. Eli reasoned that any escape, whatever it turned out to be, would have to involve one of the vehicles or they could just forget it.

As they bumped and jostled their way past Solferino they notice a few small farms and cultivated fields, and Eli felt like they must be nearing Chiquilá. Just after crossing an area of mangrove swamp the first buildings appeared ahead of them. Small houses of poor construction and a couple of small stores were all they saw as they drove towards the center of the village. What passed for a hotel was visible on their right and a few storage buildings lay ahead near the ferry landing.

"Now I see why these guys wanted to buy gas down the road," said Paco, clearly surprised by the minimal services of the town. "There's nothing in this place. Hey, old man - you sure we can do this thing here?"

"Not to worry, Paco," said Vicente wearily.

They drove down to the ferry dock, and to the right of the traffic circle they saw five large trucks with no markings parked next to the seawall.

"Look, you see this? The *Mexicanos* already bring the trucks." Vicente smiled, satisfied that the plan was working.

The drivers pulled the big SUV's in next to the trucks and everyone got out to inspect the area. There were no drivers in the trucks but they could only be there to receive the drugs, as planned. Paco, Eli, and Vicente were about to discuss the logistics of unloading the cargo when Rudy interrupted and pointed at a guy in a white suit, walking across the road towards them. Two of the guards moved quickly to block his path and the guy put his hands up to show he was unarmed. After a brief conversation, he was allowed to pass and he walked up to the group and waved.

"*Hola*. My name José Almagro. Welcome to Chiquilá. I am represent *Señor* Garcia-Puli. He is here only for five minutes to see you. Please come with me."

The brisk wind blew his wild black hair blew over his face, partly obscuring his tanned, thick features and large black mustache. He was older than he first appeared, maybe mid-forties, and his face was deeply lined and furrowed like a farmer's field.

Almagro wore a black shirt with no tie and was smiling so broadly that Eli thought there must be something wrong. He scanned the area looking for a place to find cover in case the meeting did not go well, but could find nothing viable between the buildings and the ferry landing.

The guards stayed with the Suburbans while Paco, Eli, and Vicente accompanied Almagro across the road and into a small building with a palm-thatched roof. A few tables and chairs were scattered about and it seemed like this was what passed for a bar in Chiquilá. Ten relatively young guys sat at the tables drinking soft drinks or bottled water and said nothing as the men entered. *They must be the drivers of the trucks, a two man team for each vehicle. Good plan*, Eli thought.

They followed Almagro behind the bar and through a door that led to what might have been the only air conditioned room within a hundred miles. Several large guys, obviously well-armed bodyguards stood between Eli and two older men who sat at a small table in the back of the room. One was larger than the other, thick-bodied with tousled black hair and a large mustache. He wore a black *guayabera* shirt and tan trousers and looked relaxed and comfortable as he spoke quietly to his companion. The other guy looked a bit younger and was not as heavy-set. He smiled a lot and his bushy eyebrows and thick mustache amplified his facial expressions when he spoke. His white *guayabera* and white trousers were spotless, and it looked like he'd just walked off a cruise ship on vacation.

Almagro approached the two men and spoke quietly, nodding his head in the direction of his three guests. The older man looked up and waved for them to come over to the table while the guards scrambled to find three more chairs.

"*Señores*, let me present *Don* Juan Garcia-Puli and *Don* Rafael Piscina. *Don* Juan, this is Paco Gutiérrez, Vicente Amarón, and Eli Rose. They have come from Miami to meet you and to be certain that everything goes well today."

"Welcome to Mexico," said Garcia-Puli in Spanish. "I trust your trip has gone well so far."

"*Si, Don* Juan," said Paco nervously. "Everything has been great."

"Good. I wanted to meet you to tell you personally that I am happy to do business with your people and I hope it will be the beginning of a long and profitable relationship."

Paco smiled and was about to say something else when Garcia-Puli interrupted him.

"Tell me, Paco, how are things in Miami? Business is good? I was hearing that maybe there have been some problems with your supply chain in the past few months, similar to what happened to you a few years ago."

"Well, we have had a couple of minor things but nothing to disrupt the business," said Paco as he wiped the sweat from his forehead with his handkerchief.

"That's good to hear. So, *Señor* Amarón, I understand that you are the person who has made this all possible. Tell me, how did you come to meet our friend Paco here?" Garcia-Puli leaned forward and appeared keenly interested in Vicente's answer.

He's not so trusting as Paco, thought Vicente. He knew what the *Don* was getting at.

"I am very well connected in Miami, *Don* Juan, and sometimes my connections tell me of business opportunities that would be good. But in this case, the information that was delivered to me came from friends in my homeland of Cuba, not from Paco's people, so you can feel good that there were no leaks."

"That is very interesting," said the *Don*, sitting back in his chair. "I know you will not mind if my people in Miami ask some questions about you. I would like to know more about your history, because you seem like a very competent man to me with much useful experience. Maybe you are someone I could use in my own organization."

Vicente smiled, feigning flattery.

"You are too kind, but for now I have a deal with Paco. Let's see what happens with that."

The *Don* smiled and Paco put his arm around Vicente's shoulder.

"He is my friend and a good business partner," added Paco disingenuously.

"And you, *Señor* Rose. What is your story? Why are you here?" Garcia-Puli looked at Eli with his bushy eyebrows raised in broad arcs.

Vicente interrupted before Eli could speak. "He is my business partner in all things," he said.

"I see," said the *Don* skeptically. He waved at one of the guards and whispered something to him, and the guy ran out of the bar.

"Gentlemen, I am afraid I must go now. I have pressing business in Cancún and then I must return to Reynosa. I thank you for coming here, and I hope you will come visit me soon so we can celebrate the start of our successful venture." He and Piscina stood and shook hands with Paco, Vicente, and Eli and then Garcia-Puli pulled Almagro aside for a quick word. Almagro nodded forcefully and smiled.

"*Si, Don* Juan," he said. Garcia-Puli left and Almagro turned to Paco.

"We can wait here until the ship arrives. Would you like something to drink?"

"Water," said Paco. Vicente and Eli agreed, and one of the guards walked out to the bar to get the bottles and some glasses.

"So, you are *Colombiano,* you are *Cubano,* and you are *gringo,* is that correct?"

Almagro sat down in the *Don's* chair with his hands folded on the table, as if he was conducting a job interview. The guard returned with the water and Eli realized they would have to endure some friendly but detailed questioning from their host, at least until the ship arrived.

"That is correct," Paco replied. "And how long have you worked for *Don* Juan?" Paco seemed to have his own plan, so Eli relaxed and sipped his water, ready to watch the fun.

Almagro smiled and looked at the table, reflecting on the question for a moment.

"I have known the *Don* since we were boys in Matamoros. My father was a business partner of his uncle, so we spent much time playing together on the ranch. I consider him to be one of my oldest friends.

And you, Paco. How did one so young come to such a high position in the Medellín group so quickly?"

Paco was no fool, and he knew why Almagro was asking the question.

"*Señor* Almagro, I *earned* my position by working my way up from the street. I have proven my loyalty and value to *Don* Pablo many times by delivering on my tasks. My position had nothing to do with our personal relationship."

Almagro frowned at the slight but kept his composure. His was a demeanor learned from years of practice and experience, of observing how business was transacted in his organization and capitalizing on those tactics that worked best.

"I don't mean any disrespect, *Señor* Gutiérrez. I was only curious. It seems maybe you do things differently in Colombia."

"I don't know about that," answered Paco, relaxing in his chair. "Family and friends always count for more. If you're not one of them, you just have to work that much harder to get the right people to notice you."

"And *Señor* Rose, you are somewhat of a mystery here. Where did you come from? What is your background?" Almagro's coal-black eyes stared intently at Eli, watching for anything that would suggest deceit.

"*Señor* Almagro, what makes you think I'm going to volunteer anything to you? I don't know you any more than you know me, so why don't we just stay acquaintances for now. We can always have a big heart to heart once we have regular business."

"Eli, that's no way to talk," said Paco with an angry look. "You should tell *Señor* Almagro something that will help him understand we can be trusted." Now Paco's stare matched that of Almagro's, cold and piercingly malevolent.

"I don't question *Señor* Almagro's trustworthiness, and I know he wouldn't question mine. But until we know each other better, I feel that the less we say the better off we will all be." Eli stared back at the Mexican, no hint of concern on his face.

Almagro smiled and sat back and sipped from his water glass.

"So, maybe in this case you have a point, *Señor* Rose. Maybe it is better that we don't share too much, for now. If this business does not continue for some reason it might be a good idea for us not to know too much about the other. A safe idea, it seems."

He looked into his glass as if a bug had landed at the bottom and then put it down on the table. Just as he was about to say something else one of the guards walked in from the other room and announced that a ship had radioed the ferry landing requesting permission to dock in less than an hour. It was just after one thirty and the ferry to Holbox still occupied the landing dock. It wasn't due to leave until two, so the ship would have to stay out until then.

"Can we go watch the process?" said Vicente.

"That's a good idea," said Almagro with a sigh. He got up and said, "Follow me." He rattled off orders in rapid sequence to the drivers and the remaining guards and walked out the front door of the bar like he was the "King" of Chiquilá.

Eli took off his jacket and tie and handed them to Rudy, who volunteered to take Vicente's and Paco's coats back to the Suburban as well. They walked over to the edge of the dock and watched the last few passengers load onto the ferry.

"There it is," said Paco, pointing towards the horizon.

Sure enough, the only ship in the area that big had to be theirs, and as the ferry began to motor out, the cargo ship slowly sailed in.

"Hey, guys!" yelled Almagro. The drivers ran from the bar and hopped into their trucks, waiting for the ferry to clear the dock before they backed onto concrete ramp. They backed up into a single line but left enough room for the loaded trucks to drive around the line and off the dock. Almagro's guards then barred entrance to the dock, sending the curious on their way with a brusque wave of their hands.

Chapter 25

The ship approached the ferry entrance slowly, as it was much longer than the dock and almost as wide as the basin entrance. The captain maneuvered the small coastal freighter expertly and let it drift in towards the main dock, where two local fisherman hauled the lines and tied them off. Two crew members immediately raced down the stairs and jumped onto the dock to check the lines and cross-tie everything. They waved up to the bridge and the captain cut the engines.

Rudy drove Paco and Almagro up to the ship in one of the Suburbans and Eli and Vicente followed with the rest of the team in the other.

"Vicente, I don't know when or if Rodríguez is going to get here, but if he does we'll need to stay low and get off this dock as fast as we can," Eli whispered.

"*Si*, Eli. It is a very dangerous place, I think."

Paco was already out of his vehicle and watching as the crew of the freighter began to move the pallets of cocaine with their large five ton crane. Several other members of the crew had joined him near the trucks and they talked politely with Almagro as the first pallet was secured on the dock.

Eli and Vicente walked up and watched as one of Almagro's men punctured one of the burlap sacks with a knife and tapped the powder into a small test tube. He added a few drops of clear liquid and it turned blue when it came into contact with the powder from the bag. The guy nodded and Almagro shook Paco's hand. It was the real stuff, and the deal was on. The Mexican waved at his guards and in a few seconds a white Lincoln Town Car drove onto the dock and down to meet them. The driver opened the back seat and Almagro turned to leave.

"I am flying to Mexico City tonight. Tomorrow morning we will transfer the funds from our banks to your accounts in the Cayman Islands, as you instructed. The funds will not clear for one week, during which we will test all the product for purity. I don't expect any problems."

"There won't be any," said Paco.

"From now on you will be dealing only with me. I will contact you in three weeks about the next shipment." Almagro shook Paco's hand.

"It has been a pleasure doing business with you, and I look forward to a long and successful venture between us."

As he was sitting down Eli and Vicente heard shouting coming from the head of the dock, immediately followed by gunfire. *Great timing*, thought Eli. They crouched behind the Suburban low enough for Eli to see a large group of hooded men dressed in black and wearing bullet proof vests storm the dock.

"Shit!" yelled Almagro. "You brought the PJF

down on us!" He pulled a Glock 19 9 millimeter pistol from his shoulder holster and pointed it at Paco.

"Tell me why I don't kill you right now," he said nervously, watching his guards trying to hold off the federal police.

Paco threw up his hands. "It's not me! Your people were followed! You screwed it up!" He suddenly pulled his own Glock and pointed it at Almagro's nose. They looked at each other for a second and realized that neither one had tipped the police. That only left one choice.

"Uh oh," said Eli. He pulled Vicente around the other side of the Suburban and dove for the ground in one motion as Paco and Almagro began shooting. The rounds peppered the Suburban but did not get close to Vicente or Eli, who huddled behind the engine block hoping not to be shot in the back by the advancing federal police.

"You bastards! I'll kill you," screamed Paco. He fired wildly and quickly exhausted his entire clip.

Paco crazily searched his pockets for another one but Almagro grabbed him by the shoulders and said, "Forget them. Let's go!"

One of the small fishing boats that was tied up on the outside of the ferry dock had raced over and was waiting for the Mexican. Almagro was a good planner, a skill he cultivated with Garcia-Puli and employed to his advantage throughout his career. He prided himself in planning for every contingency one could imagine, and the boat was just such a contingency, his emergency escape plan in case something went wrong.

Almagro and Paco jumped in with Paco yelling

at the top of his lungs, "I'll get you!" as the boat wheeled around and sped out towards the bay.

The shooting at the head of the dock had stopped and Eli didn't even need to turn around to know that the PJF were racing towards them, guns drawn. He pulled Vicente down to the ground again and said, "Lay face down with your hands over your head. Maybe they won't kill us right away. And don't look at anyone's face until we see Rodríguez or someone else with an FBI or DEA ID."

The two men lay there motionless as the hooded police officers advanced on them, while the crew on the ship did the same and put their hands behind their heads. Two Bell Jet Ranger 206 B-3's swooped in low and landed in front of the line of vehicles, blocking any possibility of escape. Rudy and the rest of the Miami team still had their guns at the ready, but he thought better of it once the helicopters landed. Eli looked under the Suburban and watched as Rudy threw is gun into the water and ordered the rest of the guys to do the same. He laid down on the concrete with a worried look, hands behind his head as the officers reached them.

The shouting was almost as loud as the helicopter engines as the federal police swept in. Eli and Vicente were handcuffed and pulled to their feet by the officers, who ran about securing the others as quickly as possible. As Vicente was pushed against the bullet-riddled Suburban he saw Rodríguez and Smith exit the helicopter closest to them, followed by several other agents he did not recognize.

Eli breathed a sigh of relief when he saw Rodríguez, and he guessed that the others aboard the helicopters probably belonged to the ATF or were senior PJF agents.

"Very good to see you," shouted Vicente over the roar of the Jet Ranger's turbine. "I was worry maybe you no come in time."

"What a mess," said Rodríguez as he walked up. He was wearing a large tactical vest with "FBI" emblazoned in yellow across the back, as well as a Bianchi ballistic nylon side holster. He holstered his Glock 22 and surveyed the scene, then said something to Smith while they walked over to speak with the senior PJF agent in the strike force. He waved and nodded and Rodríguez came back with one of the PJF officers, who unlocked Eli and Vicente's handcuffs.

"You guys are coming with us," he said, grabbing Vicente by the arm and pushing him towards the first helicopter. Smith escorted Eli and they sat next to each other in the back seats. One of the PJF officers closed the cabin doors and they fastened their seatbelts and put their headsets on. Rodríguez gave the pilot the signal to leave, and he cranked up the rotor speed and lifted off the dock.

The Jet Ranger circled the scene once before they left, and Eli could see the PJF officers unloading the cocaine and lining up the drivers and guards for processing and transport back to Mérida. At the head of the dock the police were going through the pockets of the dead guards and dragging their bodies into a line so they could be photographed in one gruesome group.

"We needed to get you out of there before we lost jurisdiction over you," said Rodríguez, looking over at Vicente. "It would have taken us weeks to get you back if they'd taken you into custody."

"How did you get us out without an argument?" asked Eli. "I would have thought they'd want to show us off as trophies along with the rest of the boys."

"We had an agreement in place that had them turn any US citizens over to us," said Smith. "Besides, they were running out of handcuffs and we said they could use ours." The young agent laughed and Eli just shook his head.

"So what happen here?" said Vicente. "This situation no was good. When we talk about this in Miami we agree that the idea is to capture Paco and the *Mexicanos* but now you have only the small fish."

"We can discuss that later," said Rodríguez. 'First, we need to clear Mexican air space."

Eli looked down at the verdant green jungle as they flew east towards Cancún. The whine of the engine and shaking of the cabin made it hard to concentrate, and it reminded Eli too much of his last flight in a Bell Huey UH-1N over the similarly green landscape along the Costa Rica-Nicaragua border.

He thought about Paco's threat and knew it was not something the guy just tossed out there. He'd have to find Paco and put him away before Paco did the same to Eli and Vicente, and that meant some deep digging was on the agenda when they got back to Miami.

The pilot began to speak to the tower at Cancún so the passengers were silent for the remainder of the flight. The Jet Ranger dropped low and came straight down the main runway and flew low over the taxi area to the private plane hangars. They bumped down and the pilot slowed his engine speed so that they could exit before he returned to Chiquilá. Smith and Rodríguez took off their headsets and shook hands with the pilot, while Eli and Vicente exited the helicopter. The walked over to the administration office, hunched low to avoid the slowly rotating propeller and waited for the two agents to join them.

When Rodríguez and Smith arrived the four men went into the administration building and asked the girl at the desk where they could find the American pilots.

"They are in the lounge area," she said, barely looking up from her magazine. "I will call them." She dialed a number on the old rotary telephone and said in Spanish,

"Tell the Americans there are some people out here to see them. Good, thanks." She glanced up at Rodríguez and added, "They will be right here." She smiled weakly and continued reading.

Within a minute the two pilots arrived from the lounge, one young guy, maybe in his late twenties with short red hair and the other, taller and older with close-cropped black hair.

"I'm Bailey. This is Serafino," said the red-haired DEA agent.

"Rodríguez, FBI. This is Smith." Smith smiled and they all shook hands.

"We appreciate the lift back," said Smith.

"No problem. Glad we can help out. No extra charge for the FBI this time."

"That's good to know, because with my budget you'd have to let me out at Islamorada." The agents all laughed, leaving Eli and Vicente feeling invisible.

"These guys are working with us down here - Vicente Amarón and Eli Rose. They're riding back with us."

"Ok, that's fine," said Bailey. "We ready to go?"

"Waiting on you," said Smith.

"Great. We need to do our pre-flight and let the tower know we're ready, so give us about thirty minutes to cool the plane down and get our window."

"Sure. You know where we can buy a Coke or something?"

"Ask the girl if you can go back and use the vending machine. But watch out, 'cause it eats pesos something fierce." Bailey's blue eyes crinkled when he smiled and he and Serafino walked out the back to the staging area.

Rodríguez asked the listless girl if they could use the machines and she replied, "*Si*," with about as much indifference as one can show. He led the way to the lounge and they sat down at the small card table while Smith tried to operate the vending machine.

"I'm buying. What do you want?" he asked.

"I'll take a Coke," said Rodríguez.

"Same for me," added Eli.

"I will have a coffee," said Vicente, who got up and helped himself to the ancient carafe that sat on a burner at the back of the lounge near the sink.

Eli shook his head, marveling at how his old mentor could drink coffee regardless of the outside temperature. Hot or cold, humid or dry, Vicente's first choice was always coffee. "That's all you ever drink," he said.

"Is no true," said Vicente as he carefully poured the boiling liquid into a Styrofoam cup. He added three packets of sugar and stirred it vigorously with a striped plastic spoon.

"Sometime I drink a beer. Also sometime a nice glass of red wine."

Smith banged on the machine after the first Coke did not escape as planned. Suddenly he was inundated with cans as they dropped out through the trap door at high velocity. He stepped back as the cans hit the floor and picked up a couple for his fellow agent and Eli.

"Maybe I also drink a Coke," said Vicente, amused by the unexpected bounty.

The other three men laughed and sat back to relax for the first time.

"We'll have the co-pilot send a message to the office while we're en route to pick up the rest of Paco's boys and search the house. I don't expect to see him there again after that fiasco on the dock, so we may have lost our shot at him." Smith was not happy but couldn't or wouldn't say what was really on his mind.

Rodríguez wasn't as diplomatic.

"Vicente, to answer your question from before, what went wrong was that the Mexicans wanted to make a big show of bringing down this operation, sort of a warning to the Gulf Cartel that their days of free reign are over. The problem was that they don't like to listen when it comes to planning, logistics, and tactics.

Smith shook his head.

"We heard a lot of, "This is our country and we know how to do it here. You *gringos* run things your way in Miami, we do it our way here." "And look what happened? A big screw up."

"But that's nothing new, is it?" asked Eli.

Both agents sighed. Rodríguez said, "Unfortunately, the PJF is not the most secure agency inside the Attorney General's office, but they can engineer a good media grab, that's for sure. They'll display all the foot soldiers, the weapons, and the drugs for the cameras, but it's done that way to keep the pressure off the real movers and shakers."

"You mean guys like Garcia-Puli?"

Smith, who had been only peripherally interested in the conversation up to that point was suddenly alert and stared hard at Eli.

"Yeah. What about him? Are you saying you saw him there?"

Vicente replied, "*Si*, he was there. But he leave maybe thirty minutes before you arrive."

"Son of a bitch!" said Smith. He looked at Rodríguez in disgust.

"Can you believe we missed him by thirty minutes? Holy shit but those PJF guys are something. They probably knew he was there. That's why we *putzed* around at the airport for an extra half hour." He stared at the can on the table and Rodríguez had a glazed look on his face.

"Sorry guys," said Eli with genuine concern. "We didn't mean to spoil the party."

"Don't apologize," said Rodríguez. "You guys did everything we asked. You did great. Looks like we were compromised from the beginning and there was nothing anyone could do. For us.........For us it's just a tough pill to swallow, because the task force has been working to get these guys for the last eighteen months, and we just missed them." He slammed his fist down on the table in frustration.

"Maybe we can find Paco," said Vicente. "He no leave Miami. He have too much business there. I believe we can find him."

"We'll see," said Rodríguez. "But you guys will need to lay low for a while until we either catch him or we can be sure he's gone. There's no doubt he'll kill you if he can find you first."

"Maybe that's what needs to happen," said Eli. "Maybe that's how we catch him - we lure him out into the open so we can grab him when he tries to move on us."

"No way," said Smith. "We can't ask you to act as bait and we can't support it. I don't think the DEA or ATF would back this, either."

Rodríguez didn't answer immediately, seeming to be lost in thought. "I don't know. It sounds too risky, but it could work."

"*Si*, this can work," added Vicente. "Paco, he want to look you in the face before he kill you so he must be there personally. When he arrive, we grab him!" He clenched his hands emphatically to add to his point.

"We'll have about two hours to talk it over on the ride back. If Smith and I can sell a plan to our superiors then we might be able to get the support we need from the other agencies. But we don't want to involve the locals. We can't afford to end up with another fiasco like this one today."

The four men sat silently for a second and the girl from the front desk knocked on the door and stuck her head in.

"The pilot say he is ready to go. You leave now."

They dropped their cans in the trash and walked out to the dark gray unmarked Beechcraft Super King Air B300C that was sitting on the inner taxiway near the building. The pilot had started the turbo's but only the propeller on the right wing was turning. They got in and the co-pilot, Serafino, pulled the stairway door up and secured it.

"Ok, guys. Seat belts fastened and no moving around until we give you clearance. Then you can grab a beer from the refreshment center and relax." He went forward and Eli relaxed for the ride back.

The plane taxied to the end of the runway and then sped away, pulling up after only a few seconds. Eli dozed as they flew over the deep blue waters of the eastern Gulf of Mexico, and away from the failed mission to capture the cartel leaders.

Chapter 26

"It's ten o'clock. Wake up, old man." Eli shook Vicente by the shoulder until he opened his eyes. "We need to get moving. I don't want to be a target any longer than I have to."

Vicente stretched and sat up, rubbing his thin hair with both hands. "I sleep on the couch all the night?" he asked.

"You were there all night, but I can't say if you were asleep or not. I was unconscious most of the night."

"I no like this idea," said the older man as he got up, headed for the bathroom. He paused, realizing that his last comment could have been misinterpreted.

"What I mean to say is you no have to do this for me. I ready to go back to my place."

Eli smiled and shook his head. "Listen old friend, Paco knows where you live and his guys will be watching your place for sure. He doesn't know anything about my background, so we're safe here, at least for a little while longer. You're staying here, and that's final."

Vicente shook his head and ambled off to the bathroom. Eli smiled and unlocked the safe behind one of the drawers in the center island of his kitchen. He retrieved his spare Beretta 92F and three loaded clips, and a Ruger .357 snub nose revolver with his extra box of hollow point rounds. *Sure hope we don't need these,* he thought as he closed up the safe and replaced the drawer.

The plan Eli and Vicente had worked out with the FBI was simple but extremely dangerous. They would return to Paco's place to reclaim Vicente's Corvette, then cruise by his apartment to be sure and give anyone watching those locations a good view of them. Since the Corvette already had an RFID transponder attached to it, the task force could follow the two men around and be within striking distance if anything happened.

However, Eli had no intention of just riding around Miami and waiting for Paco to take pot shots at him. That could take days or weeks, if it even happened at all. Everyone guessed that Paco was back in town, mainly because the Miami operation was so critical to the Medellín Cartel's marketing plan, but he was likely under deep cover, and only a clear path to his betrayers would flush him out into the open.

It took some effort, but Eli persuaded Vicente to use Julio and his connections to make the contact. Vicente didn't know if Julio would help them again, but he bet that he would, since things had gone so well in Pinar de Río.

He emerged from the bathroom looking polished and alert, considering he'd been in the same clothes for two days and hadn't slept in a decent bed. Eli handed him the .357 and the box of hollow points and said,

"Just in case, Ok *amigo*? I don't want anything happening to you."

The older man smiled and looked at the weapon.

"Is very nice of you, Eli. Very nice."

"Ok, let's go get the Corvette, then we'll run by your place so you can see what's happened to it. You can pick up some extra clothes and whatever else is worth salvaging and then we'll make some calls."

They called a Yellow Cab and arrived at Paco's former home amidst a tangle of Orchid task force vehicles and law enforcement officers. After some discussion with a highly suspicious FBI agent at the front gate, Eli and Vicente were permitted to enter with an escort to talk to Rodríguez for a minute.

The Special Agent saw them walking in and went to meet them, smiling from behind his sunglasses.

"Vicente, Eli, good to see you. How do you feel?"

"I Ok," answered Vicente. "We come to start the plan. We take the car and go to my place now."

The smile dropped from the young Special Agent's face. "You sure about this? We're ready to go, but I still don't like the plan very much."

"We're ready," replied Eli. "This is better than just waiting to get picked off one day, six months from now. We need to get this guy to move aggressively, so let's get on with it."

Rodríguez waved at another agent who was talking in a group near a large white panel van. He ran over and Rodríguez introduced him.

"This is Special Agent Farrell. He and his team will be in the van and will monitor your location at all times. They will also have a couple of transmitters for your clothes, just in case you're out of the car and something happens. Smith and I will follow in one of our vehicles and will be in radio contact with the van so we can be ready to make the bust. Any questions?"

"Nope," said Eli.

"Ok, then. Please go with Agent Farrell and he'll set you up with the microphones."

They walked over to the van and Farrell introduced the two men to his team.

"Guys, meet Vicente and Eli. They're our "pigeons" for this operation. Let's get 'em wired up so we can get this show on the road."

Farrell smiled broadly and flipped a thick lock of blond hair off his forehead. His college-boy good looks and brilliant smile belied his history as an ex-Navy Seal and weapons specialist, and he used that to great advantage when he worked under cover. He was constantly underestimated by friends and foes alike, and that led to a successful arrest record and a series of early promotions. He was a guy on the rise, and had been picked as an early candidate for advancement by his superiors in the FBI. Even Rodríguez recognized that his young subordinate would soon pass him by.

Eli and Vicente were fitted with microphones and small transmitters inside their shirts and following a few minutes of testing, were escorted to the Corvette by Farrell.

"We'll be monitoring everything that happens, so if the guy jumps ya' we'll be there in thirty seconds," he said.

"Better be faster than that," added Eli. "I don't think

he wants to give us a big hug when he sees us. More likely he'll shoot first and ask questions later."

Farrell smiled. "We'll be there in time," he said.

They all shook hands and Eli and Vicente drove out through the gate, leaving the task force to their work at the compound. They soon arrived at Vicente's apartment complex and parked in his spot. He looked up at his window but could see nothing through the lowered shade.

"Now we see," he said to Eli as they climbed the stairs to the front door. Vicente turned the knob and the door opened, a clear sign that someone had been there. They pulled their weapons and cautiously opened the door, wary of any motion inside. Vicente entered slowly and saw no one, so he put the .357 back in his belt and stood there staring forlornly at his wrecked place.

"Good thing you don't collect paintings or ceramics," said Eli somewhat morosely. "They pretty much trashed the place."

Vicente sighed and began to pick up the furniture and clothes from the floor. "Yes, is no good what they do."

Eli hugged his old mentor and patted him on the back. "Sorry, old friend. I know things like this are tough."

"No worry. As you say, I no collect things so is only clothes. I get a bag, then we go."

Vicente wandered off slowly into his bedroom and returned after a few minutes with a suit bag and small overnight bag stuffed with clothes and toiletries. They were about to leave when the telephone rang, startling both men.

"You know who that is?" said Eli.

Vicente picked up the receiver and said, "Hello. *Si.* I understand. *Si,* we do it right now." The look on his face was grave, and he looked drained by the conversation.

"They have Rita," he said coldly.

"How's that possible?" said Eli loudly. "I sent her to Orlando days ago to visit her sister. They can't know where she lives."

"I don know, but Paco want to do a trade - me for Rita. He say he kills her in four hours unless we do the deal." Vicente sat down on the edge of his overturned sofa with his head hung low.

"I just don't believe it," said Eli. "It's got to be a trick. Let's check her place and then the office, just to be sure."

They left Vicente's place quickly and drove to Rita's condominium building to see if she might still be in town. Her little red Mazda Miata was still in her parking place but that didn't bother Eli too much. *She would have flown,* he thought. They checked the door to her place and it was locked; there was no sign of forced entry or any other sign she had been kidnapped.

"Let's check the office, just to be sure," said Eli.

When they arrived it was instantly clear what had happened. Rita must have ignored Eli's order to leave immediately, maybe intending to finish off some work and close up the office on Friday as usual. The office door was ajar and the Rita's desk had been turned over onto the floor. The other offices had been ransacked as well; the place was a shambles.

"They must have grabbed her at the end of the day on Friday," said Eli. "Probably just enough time for them to get here before she closed up. Didn't you say they had no idea about the office?"

"There is no way they know about this," said Vicente with anger. "They don know. How this happen, Eli?"

"They must have blown your cover sometime during the week and been watching the place. Maybe they didn't grab you because they needed to see how the deal would work in Cuba first. Paco must have called his guys here when he got back to Mérida. That's the only way I can explain it."

Vicente grabbed a handful of hair and said, "Eli, what we do now?"

"Was it Paco that you spoke to on the phone back at your apartment?"

"No. Is one of his guys - Alvaro, I think."

Eli thought for a second. "Paco will want to set up the exchange in someplace he knows very well, someplace he can control. Where do you think he'd want to do this?"

"Along the river," answered Vicente without hesitation. "Maybe in the same place we do the first meeting."

"Ok. Call Julio. Explain the situation to him and tell him we need to find Paco and get a message to him that you'll do the deal tonight. Farrell, I hope you guys got that," Eli said, hoping the task force agents could hear their plan.

Vicente nodded and picked the telephone up off the floor and called Julio. The argument was heated and there was no shortage of threats launched by Vicente, but in the end Julio relented and agreed to help. If the end result was that Paco was put away or disposed of, it worked for him. But if Paco got away, Vicente knew the consequences. It would be his head on the chopping block of his old comrades in arms, and they wouldn't hesitate to dispose of him as a nuisance who'd lost his value. So much for brotherhood.

"We must wait here for one hour," said Vicente as he tried to calm down. "Julio makes the call and tell them to call us here. Then we see what he do."

Eli turned over Rita's chair and dragged one in from his office.

"Well then, take a seat and relax. We'll just have to wait."

He wondered if Farrell and his team had heard what was planned and would be there in enough time when things got nasty to bail them out. He doubted it.

The telephone rang less than forty five minutes after he spoke with Julio.

"*Si*, said Vicente. "*Si, si*, I understand. No police. Is Ok. We will be there." He hung up and rubbed his face. "In the same place as before - the parking lot where Northwest North River Drive run into Southwest 3rd Street. Seven in the night for the trade and we no can be late."

"Ok, don't worry," said Eli. "Let's make sure our FBI friends got all this."

Eli left the office and went down to the parking garage to look for Farrell and the van but saw nothing. He considered calling Rodríguez right then but decided to wait until they had to leave for the meeting with Paco. Instead, he went back up to the office and placed a call to Jim Morgan at home.

§

"Just a minute," said Morgan's wife, a bit irritated.

"Jim," she called out, "you have a call. Someone named Eli Rose. He says it's important." She paused to listen for a second and said to Eli, "He says he'll be right with you."

"Thanks very much," said Eli.

The telephone was put down on a table or some other hard surface for nearly a minute while Eli waited in silence.

"Ok," said Morgan, suddenly breaking in. "What's so important that you have to call me at home on a Saturday afternoon?"

"Jim, we've had some problems down here and I need some information."

"You know I can't help you with anythin'," said Morgan. "But tell me what's goin' on and I'll see what I can do."

"Paco Gutiérrez got away," Eli began, "and he somehow knew about Vicente's connection to the office. He's kidnapped Rita and wants to trade her for Vicente."

"Aw, shit. That's too bad about Rita, but you know I can't put shoes on the street for you."

"I know that. What I really need to know is if the Coast Guard caught the sub."

"No," said Morgan with a sigh. "They were waitin' for 'em in international waters but whoever commands that thing really knows his stuff. They stayed in Cuban territorial waters until they were south of Pinar del Rio and then continued along the southern coast until they got to Cienfuegos. That was where things got strange."

"How so?"

"They actually went into the bay and tied up at one of the long refinery docks. They're still there, from what we can see from the Blackbird photos. There are no facilities for 'em so we can't figure out what they're doin'. The cutter that was trackin' 'em put into Guantanamo, so it's a stalemate for now."

"Did they try and communicate with anyone?" Eli asked.

"Not as far as we can tell," said Morgan. "No radio or other transmission from 'em at all."

"That's good. Maybe I can use that when we meet with Paco. One last thing - any rumblings from the usual grapevines about DEA or FBI agents on the take down here?"

There was silence for a few seconds, as if Morgan was considering what to say before he spoke.

"You know how the chatter works," he said. "You hear things from time to time. Most of it is garbage, tough to sort through in many ways. But you do hear things."

"Clue me in."

Morgan sighed audibly. "Ok, so there are rumors floatin' around about a federal agent who may be in the pocket of the drug cartels. Nothin' firm, no names, just this persistent rumor. You might want to watch yourself down there."

Great, Eli thought. *Now you tell me.* "Thanks for the words of wisdom."

"Take care, Eli. We still have some work to do, and I'd hate to have to find someone else."

"Morgan, you are such a caring guy. I appreciate it."

"Sure, no problem. Talk to you soon."

"Yeah, I hope so," said Eli. He felt abandoned again by The Agency, and couldn't trust any of the agents he'd been dealing with at the FBI or DEA. He might have to make a call on who in the task force he could trust, and that was little more than a hunch and a gamble at this point. He hoped he chose well.

Before he shared his suspicions with Vicente, Eli decided to call Bill Sexton and make good on his earlier promise.

"Bill, it's Eli. I promised to give you something on this case before it wrapped up, so you better be listening and have a pen and paper ready."

"Sure, Eli, I'm ready. Fire away."

"Before I tell you I just want you to know that what's going to happen may be pretty ugly, so you should plan on keeping a safe distance. Vicente and I have a meeting with Paco Gutiérrez at seven tonight in the parking lot where Northwest North River Drive connects with Southwest 3rd Street. I'm expecting things to flare up and there may be some shooting, so be forewarned."

"Eli, when has anything you've ever done not been

dangerous or involved a gunfight of some type?"

Eli laughed and had to agree with his old friend.

"Ok, so you already know the drill. I'd just feel bad if something happened and I hadn't warned you first."

"Understood," said Sexton, "and thanks for keeping your end of the deal."

"Don't mention it," Eli added. "Hope I don't see you there."

He hung up and considered what to tell Vicente. He felt Vicente should know about the mole in the Orchid task force because he might be able to guess who it was, but the rest wasn't important for now. Eli walked into what was left of Vicente's office and dragged a chair up off the floor.

"Vicente, I just got off the phone with Jim in Virginia. He said there are rumors floating around that one of our task force guys is on the take from the cartels."

"My God," exclaimed Vicente. "If this true then is an explanation for why they know about the office.. I so sorry, Eli. I trust this guys."

"I know, old friend. We can't do anything about it now, but I want you to think back and tell me if you can put your finger on a likely mole. Do you suspect anyone."

Vicente sat back and rubbed his chin, remembering what had taken place between he and the agents over the past few days. "I no can tell who is the guy," he said slowly. "But I think this kid Rodríguez is Ok. I trust him."

That was good enough for Eli. Vicente had been his teacher and had probably forgotten more about how to read someone than Eli ever knew. He decided to call Rodríguez and tell him about the meeting near the Miami River and what was at stake.

"This is Rodríguez. How can I help you?"

"This is Eli. The meeting is going down in a parking lot at Northwest North River Drive and Southwest 3rd Street. They want to exchange Vicente for my assistant. Seems like they grabbed her sometime Friday. We're on our way in a few minutes, so make sure your team is on us. I haven't seen a trace of them."

"Ok, thanks for telling me," said Rodríguez with concern. "What do you mean you haven't seen my guys? They must just be keeping a low profile. You must have missed them."

"I don't think so," replied Eli, "but I don't have time to worry about them now. Just make sure you stay with us."

"We'll do what we can to support you," said the young Special Agent, "but our primary objective is to take down Gutiérrez, you understand that?"

"Sure, I understand," Eli answered. "But maybe you could place a sharpshooter or two on the overpass or near one of the buildings at the back of the parking lot."

"Like I said, Eli, we'll do what we can."

"Thanks," said Eli. "Oh, and by the way, next time you might want to choose your team carefully."

"What does that mean?" The tone of Rodríguez' voice changed noticeably and not positively.

"Rumor has it that one of your people is on the take. Unless you want another operation blown I would be careful about who you involve in this one."

Eli's comment was answered by silence, which he

supposed meant that he'd just said something he shouldn't have. But he was surprised by Rodríguez' reply.

"Ok, good point. I'll think about it. Thanks for trusting me with that."

"Sure. We'll be looking for you and your guys to come riding in like the cavalry when we make the exchange, so don't disappoint me," Eli said, hopefully.

"We'll be there. Good luck."

That was the best he could do under the circumstances, but Eli still felt like they might be mostly on their own. He told Vicente what Rodríguez had said and how he reacted to the warning about a mole.

"What you think, Eli? He dirty or he Ok?"

"Well, *Papi*, if I learned any of what you taught me about such things, I'd have to say he's clean. I guess we'll find out for sure tonight." Vicente nodded and Eli added, "Let's review how we want this to go so that we have some contingencies planned out."

The two men planned as best they could how they would try and manage the meeting with Paco and his men. Vicente would take Rita's place but no one intended for him to leave with Paco. Eli would make sure Rita was safe before they acted. Despite the RFID tracking unit, they'd have to take Eli's car because it was larger and made of steel and not fiberglass, like Vicente's old Corvette. It would offer at least some protection if the bullets started flying.

Vicente would stand right next to the car so that when Paco's men surrounded him he would have some space between himself and the guy behind him. If everything went the way they hoped, Eli would put Rita on the ground or under the car if there was time so that when the shooting started she was out of the direct line of fire. Vicente had to rely on his reflexes and his ability to separate himself from his captors so that Eli could get off a shot, if needed. That would be the hairiest part of the plan, as they were sure that Paco wanted them in the open, with no cover. Eli just hoped that any shooting would be from panicked guys who were poor shots anyway, and that none of the wounds they were sure to suffer would be fatal.

They both decided they couldn't wait for Rodríguez and his people to move first, so they would do what they could. They removed their microphones and transmitters and Vicente handed Eli back his .357.

"I'll give it back when I can," Eli said. He slipped the weapon into his trousers.

"It's almost time, my friend. Are you ready for this?"

"*Si*, of course. I always ready for thing like this," said the older man with a smile. Even though Vicente seemed relaxed and confident, Eli knew he was contemplating a bad outcome.

"Eli, one more thing. If this no go so well, you know what to do, *Si*?"

"If you mean I have to get Rita out Ok, you don't have to say it. You can count on it - she'll be fine. But don't worry because nothing's going to happen to you, either." Eli patted his mentor on the shoulder and smiled.

"Everyone goes home Ok tonight, old friend."

Vicente just smiled but didn't answer. Eli looked at his watch and said, "We better get into position. Let's go."

They left the office and headed down to the garage to get Eli's GTO. They drove down Brickell Avenue and turned on Southwest 7th Street, headed for the bridge over the Miami River on Southwest 2nd Avenue. As Eli made the turn onto 7th he noticed a large white panel van make the same turn, and realized that Farrell and his team were tailing them at a safe distance.

"I see Special Agent Farrell and his guys have spotted us," said Eli.

Vicente turned around in his seat to look.

"Maybe is a good thing. Maybe is the team Rodríguez pick to get Paco."

Eli looked back into the rear-view mirror and shook his head. "I don't know," he replied. "It doesn't feel right to me."

He turned on Southwest 2nd Avenue and crossed the bridge, then turned left on Southwest 3rd Street and headed for the parking lot under the I-95 overpass. Eli surveyed the scene as they drove up and Paco's men were already there, the two black Chevy Suburbans parked at either end of the lot. Other than some scrub bushes behind them, there were no obvious places of concealment where Rodríguez' FBI team could cover them and he didn't see any signs of marksmen on the overpass, not that they could get a clear shot off from that angle anyway.

I guess Farrell is the guy, he thought. *I hope he moves his ass when the fun starts.*

Chapter 27

Eli pulled in and parked at an angle between the two SUV's. They were far enough away that the drivers decided to move closer, and drove up to box them in from either end. No one got out of the vehicles until they could see the black Mercedes approaching from Northwest North River Drive. It stopped directly in front of but perpendicular to the GTO, nose in but with enough space so that Vicente would have to walk across to it in the open.

Paco's men got out, a new crew of eight young guys sporting handguns and late model Mac-10's with suppressors. The men stood in front of their vehicles and formed an arc around the GTO, but no one walked in behind them, which Eli was relieved to see. That meant that he could throw Rita under the car when things got really bad and she would be somewhat out of the action there. He and Vicente opened their doors and got out but didn't walk away from the car.

"Paco," Eli called out. "We're here. Let's get this thing over with."

The back doors of the big Mercedes jerked open

and Paco got out on Eli's right, and one of his men exited to his left holding Rita by the arm.

"So, I see that son of a bitch Vicente is with you. I'm surprised he had the guts to come. What did you have to do, put a gun to his head?"

Paco looked surprisingly good, especially considering the fact that his place had been overrun by the task force and he'd surely lost most of his extensive wardrobe. He wore a white three piece suit with white shoes and a white belt, and a dark blue shirt open at collar down to his chest. He took off his sunglasses and smiled, but Eli knew he wasn't happy.

"Paco, let's cut to the chase. You offered the girl for Vicente, and he's willing to do it. Are you?" Vicente moved a step forward but Eli subtly grabbed his sleeve to hold him back.

"Sure, Eli. A deal's a deal. You know, you guys could have been rich if you just followed through with the plan. I don't get it - why'd you turn on me?" The kid seemed genuinely hurt, and Vicente remembered how well he'd treated his old team. Paco valued loyalty and gave it in return, but you could never trust a drug dealer and Vicente knew this from the beginning.

"Because you are no good," he shouted back before Eli could answer. Eli shot his old mentor a dirty look, but Vicente didn't care. He was ready to get the business over with.

"Send over the girl," Eli called out. "When she's safe Vicente will come over."

Paco laughed. "You think so? How about Vicente comes first and then we send the girl?"

"No dice. She goes first or no deal."

Paco contemplated the plan for a second and then mumbled something to the guy holding Rita by the arm. She pulled herself free and Paco nodded, letting her walk over to Eli and Vicente. Paco's men braced for action as she walked slowly towards her friends, being careful not to go too slow or too fast. As she approached, Eli noticed that the same guy that let her go had opened the trunk of the Mercedes and handed Paco a large stainless steel briefcase.

Rita was clearly scared but she stayed composed, and Vicente hugged her and asked her in Spanish if she was Ok. She nodded weakly, so he pushed her behind him and in tightly next to the car.

"You listen to Eli," he said, and she nodded again. Eli saw that she looked tired but otherwise unharmed, and he was relieved to see that Paco at least had stayed away from her.

Vicente was about to walk out into the open when Paco suddenly threw the briefcase across the parking lot towards them. It came to a sliding stop a few feet away and the trio fell into a crouch as if it was about to explode.

"See you around, Eli," Paco called out as he got back into the Mercedes. His men suddenly lowered their weapons and got into their SUV's. Eli glanced over his shoulder and saw the large white FBI panel van coming towards them at high velocity. The Mercedes and the Suburbans raced off down Northwest North River Drive before the van arrived and disappeared under the overpass.

"They must have spotted the "Fed's," said Eli as the van screeched to a stop in front of the GTO. He hugged

Rita and smiled, and Vicente visibly sagged against the car with relief.

Farrell and team jumped out of the van with their guns drawn, looking around for the drug dealer and his men.

"You missed the party," said Eli as the young agent approached them. "They just took off that way. If you go now you might be able to catch them."

There were two junior agents and a young female agent with Farrell, all wearing body armor. They paused and stayed behind as Farrell approached, but did not holster their weapons.

"Is that so?" said Farrell. "Too bad about that. Well, what do we have here?" He reached down and picked up the scuffed briefcase, holding it up for Eli and Vicente to see.

"I have no idea," Eli replied. "Paco just threw it at us before he left. We haven't had a chance to open it yet."

"Well let's just see what's inside." Farrell put the briefcase on the hood of the GTO and opened it, rotating it around so the other three could see the contents.

"Interesting, very interesting."

"What the hell?" said Eli, astonished. Vicente and Rita also stared wide-eyed at the contents of the briefcase, which was filled with stacks of hundred dollar bills.

"Looks like a lot of cash here, Eli. What would ya' say - fifty thousand - no one hundred thousand dollars? Yeah, that seems about right. Looks to me like a payoff for something, maybe for helping him get away in

Mexico. Yeah, I bet that's it. It's a payoff for your help blowing our bust in Mexico." Farrell brushed a lock of blond hair off his forehead and smiled at the trio.

"Hey, wait just a second," Eli stammered. "There's no way we helped him escape. Rodríguez knows - we were working with you guys from the beginning. This is a set up." Vicente nodded and Rita looked on nervously.

"Maybe, maybe not." The young agent closed the briefcase and held it in his left hand. With his right hand he leveled his Glock 22 at Eli and added, "What do ya' think an inquest would say about this? Hey Ruthy, what do ya' think IA will say about this?"

His young assistant smiled and walked up behind him with her gun pointed at Vicente.

"I think it's pretty clear that they were bought off by Gutiérrez and we just happened to catch them before they got away with the cash."

"Yep, that's what it looks like to me, too," said Farrell. "Too bad they wouldn't cooperate and surrender when we caught 'em in the act, isn't it?" The other two agents moved in and grabbed Vicente and Eli by the arms and started pulling them towards the van.

"Just a big shame they decided to put up a fight. If there was any other way, we would have taken them alive, but it's too bad they decided to shoot it out with us."

Rita looked around, panic-stricken and said, "Eli, what's happening?"

"Shut up, sister," shouted Ruth as she grabbed and shoved Rita towards the van.

"Stay cool," Eli said.

"Good plan," added Farrell. "That just makes everything easier for all of us. Just get in the van." He pointed the gun at Eli's face and the group walked off to the back of the vehicle. Ruth handed Rita off to Farrell and opened the back so they could get in.

"Cuff 'em first. We don't want any games while we're driving. That would be dangerous."

The other two agents handed over their handcuffs and Ruth jerked Eli's hands behind his back and cuffed him before he got into the van. She did the same for Vicente and Rita, then got in with one of the other agents and sat next to them on the short metal benches that lined each side. Farrell slammed the door shut and got into the driver's side, while his other agent drove Eli's GTO.

"Where you take us?" said Vicente.

"Never mind that," hissed Ruth. She flipped her hair around when she looked at Vicente and her blond pony tail smacked Eli in the nose.

"Sit quietly and we'll have a nice, peaceful ride."

The van started off and swerved around dangerously, giving everyone the impression that it might flip on its side at the next sharp curve. Soon, however, they were running on smooth pavement and cruising at a high rate of speed.

"They're taking us down Kendall Drive out past Krome Avenue," guessed Eli. "They're going to finish us out there and plant the money on us, then call it in like it just happened." Ruth and the other agent glared at Eli but said nothing, so he continued.

"They will plant some weapons on us and shoot

some holes in a few things to make it look like we put up a fight. Then we'll all get a severe case of lead poisoning from these nice new Glocks they're holding, and poof, problem solved."

Ruth nodded at her compatriot and he hit Eli hard in the stomach with the butt of his pistol. Eli groaned and struggled to breath, while Rita started to sob into Vicente's shoulder.

"Shut up!" yelled the girl.

Her blue eyes flashed in anger as she moved to hit Rita with her gun. Vicente rose up to block the blow and succeeded, catching the gun butt on his left cheek. It opened a small gash and blood streamed down his face and neck onto his shirt. He winced and sat back, but was satisfied with his sacrifice.

Rita stopped sobbing and cowered next to Vicente, who sat upright and defiant.

"Cut the crap," said the young male agent. "We don't want to have to explain shit like this to IA." He frowned at his partner and she sat back, bumping her head against the side of the van.

"You're right," said Ruth, rubbing the sore spot. "Sorry - wasn't thinking. So yeah, wise guy, we have a nice aggregate pond for you to visit out past Krome. You've got a pretty good imagination, I'll give you that much. Pretty much nailed it dead on. You feel better now, knowing what's going to happen?"

"Not really," gasped Eli, still trying to catch his breath. "But thanks for being honest about it. So what are you getting out of this? The money? Doesn't seem like much."

Both of the agents laughed and Ruth said, "This?

This is chicken feed, it's nothing. We're sacrificing this to make it look good."

"So how much?"

Eli believed that if he could get her to talk and engage with them, she might hesitate just enough when it came time to pull the trigger to allow him to do something. What, he didn't know, but it was better than just sitting by silently, waiting for the inevitable.

"You're not on the need to know list," she said with a smile. "Anyway, it's a helluva' lot more than this." She kicked the briefcase like it was worthless.

"Why you do this?" Vicente added. "Why you take the money from this guy? Is no worth it."

Ruth stretched her legs out across the van but held her pistol tightly. She smiled and said, "You can't pass it up. There's just *so* much money. Every day we see millions and millions of dollars rolled up in these busts, and all it does is go back to some dirty politicians in Washington so they can steal it while no one is looking. Why shouldn't we have a share? We're the one's risking our necks out here to protect and serve, not them. They just sit around and suck the life out of.........."

"Can it!" shouted her partner. "Don't tell these assholes anything else. Since you're just venting you can keep it between us." He shot her an angry stare and she looked away momentarily.

"So, what about it? They're dead anyway, and it makes me feel good to get it off my chest." Ruth paused and when her partner said nothing, she continued as if she was in confession.

"So now we get something for risking it every day for all you simple folks. In another year I'll be able to retire and really enjoy life for a change."

"Yeah, what will you do? What are your plans?" Eli kept trying to pull her out, and slowly his plan was working.

Ruth turned toward him slightly and looked at him quizzically.

"Why do you care?"

"Well, I'm a short-timer as far as I can tell, and maybe it just makes me think about what could have been for me if I hear you talk about how you're going to spend the money. That's all."

The girl reflected on his question for a second and said, "I'm buying an island somewhere in the Pacific. I'm gonna' build a nice place on a hill overlooking a quiet bay, someplace that catches the breezes no matter what time of the year it is. I'll lay on the sand and swim in the ocean and just let the world do whatever the hell it wants to, just without me."

"I'm envious," said Eli. "Even in my wildest dreams I could never have done something like that. I can see why you were tempted."

Both agents looked at him somewhat surprised but without comment. Vicente sensed an opening and he jumped in aggressively.

"So what it takes to stop this?"

"What?" said Ruth.

"I say, what it take to change the plan, no to kill us?"

Ruth looked at her partner for a second, then said, "Why? How much have you got?"

"Kowalski, what the hell did Farrell say about talking to these losers? Can the chit chat, now!"

"Screw you, Pike," shouted Ruth at her red-faced partner. "Why shouldn't we check out the competition? Not like there's another big payday in it for us after this job. Maybe we can get a bonus before we're done."

"That's not the plan," said Pike. "We go with the plan. That's the way Farrell set it up with the Colombians, and that's what we're gonna' do."

"Why should we always do it his way?" she answered. "Because Farrell get's a bigger cut, that's why, and he gets his rocks off whenever he wants with that little Cuban whore of his. I think it's time we started getting some action of our own."

Ruth was mad and focused on winning her argument rather than on her prisoners, so she didn't notice the light tap that Rita's handcuff's made as they fell onto the bench behind her. Even though she often presented herself as a tough as nails, no nonsense type of girl, Rita was actually small and thin-boned, and with a bit of effort she was able to slip out of Ruth's handcuffs without being noticed. She touched Vicente's hands and he knew instantly that she was free, but she kept her hands behind her back so that no one was the wiser.

Pike looked at the floor and said nothing, but Eli suspected he was considering his options. Any move to do something other than what was planned would have negative consequences for both of them, but the two agents clearly weren't satisfied with the status quo and Vicente seemed to have provided exactly the right catalyst for the occasion.

"Vicente," asked Eli, "tell them how much we can lay our hands on, right now."

Both agents looked at Vicente with keen interest. He answered, "We have ten million dollars," he lied. "How much it take to save us?"

Ruth looked at Pike and then looked back at Vicente and smiled. "You pay us eight million and you're free as a bird. You can do that?"

Vicente protested. "Is most of the money. Is no fair."

"You wanna' bargain?" said Ruth incredulously. "Are you serious?"

Eli kicked Vicente in the shin so that everyone could see, so he shook his head vigorously. "Ok, is a deal. Is no problem for us."

"You know what'll happen if you're lying just to get out of here?" said Pike. "We'll pick you up again, only the next time there won't be any negotiation."

"We get it," Eli chimed in. "But why do you think Gutiérrez wants us out of the picture so badly? I'll answer that for you - so that we don't force him out of his own gig. I just came back from a visit with Manuel Durán in Trinidad, and we got along real well. I can slip right into the same space as Paco, and Paco knows it. That's why this is going on. And let me tell you something else. We'll pay better than Paco. He's taking you guys for granted because he gives the big bucks to Farrell. You're just chaff to him, something he can replace whenever he wants."

"Big talk," said Pike still staring at the floor. "Why should we believe any of this?"

"Because you know I'm right."

Pike paused again before he spoke, but this time he stared directly at Eli.

"Rodríguez said you guys were working for us, for the FBI. How do we know you're not just blowing smoke up our skirts?"

Eli answered immediately and with conviction. "Let me ask you something, Agent Pike. The FBI picks you up on the street and threatens you with the full weight of federal prosecution, like they did with Vicente. So what are *you* going to do? You'll cut a deal, whatever you can get, that's what. Sure, we both worked with your guys in Mexico; hell, why wouldn't we, considering the alternatives. But if you ask Smith and Rodríguez how they got onto us in the first place they'll tell you it was because Vicente was making a deal with Paco to trans-ship coke through Cuba to Mexico. Now, does that sound like we're government stooges?"

Ruth looked at Pike and then at Eli.

"Listen up," she began slowly. "You follow my lead. When I say jump, you jump. When I say run, you run like hell. And see that your tootsie here get's her ass in gear or we'll leave her behind."

Rita shot the girl a dirty look but stayed quiet.

"We'll take care of Farrell and Hunter and plant the cash on them. We'll testify to the fact that Paco had them bought and paid for and they tried to get us to go along."

"We had no choice," added Pike, seemingly in a better mood. "They forced us to fire, so we took 'em down. It might get hot for awhile," he looked at Ruth, "but we'll skate."

"Don't worry about us," Eli replied. "We're highly motivated to get out of this, so we'll do whatever you say."

Ruth smiled slightly and looked away. Pike stared into space, not seeming to focus on anything in particular. Eli looked at Vicente, who winked his blood-stained eye to acknowledge the plan.

The van soon turned off Kendall Drive and bumped along a gravel-packed access road to one of the many limestone aggregate plants that form the tenuous border between the burgeoning city and the Everglades. No one worked on Saturdays so the place would be deserted, a perfect location for the day's events. The air conditioning stopped working in the back of the van and the space began to heat up like an oven in the late afternoon sun.

Eli considered himself fortunate that the ride was almost over, as he knew that the longer they drove, the more chance there was of his two captors changing their minds. The van slid to a stop and Eli could hear the GTO drive up next to them, the hard limestone crunching under its tires.

Farrell open the back of the van and shouted, "Out! Come on, let's go."

Ruth jumped out first and backed up a few feet, holding her Glock on the trio. Eli climbed out next and Rita stayed close to him, hoping to hide the fact that she was free of the handcuffs she held in her hands. Vicente closed up tightly behind her, trying to shield her hands from view. The tactic worked because Pike did not notice anything unusual as he followed them out. They stood there staring silently at Farrell.

"Time's up," he said with a grin. "Pike, ya' got the briefcase?" Pike held it up for him to see. "Good." He nodded at Ruth, who moved to take off their handcuffs. "We need ya' to fall naturally and those handcuffs won't let that happen. Ya' don't mind, do ya'?"

Eli rubbed his wrists and said, "No argument from me."

Ruth moved over behind Rita and froze, seeing that she'd removed her handcuffs.

"Is there a problem?" Farrell said.

"No, everything's Ok," Ruth answered, still somewhat shaken. She pretended to remove Rita's handcuffs but instead grabbed them and threw them to Pike. She moved over to Vicente and removed his handcuffs and tossed them to Farrell.

"Ok, we finally ready here?" said Farrell. "Good," he continued, not waiting for their answer. "Let's see. Hunter, please escort Eli here to the driver's side of his car. Let's have him found on the ground with the front door open."

Hunter grabbed Eli by the arm but Eli threw him off. He walked over without "assistance" and stood by the open car door.

"Pike, take Vicente here to the other door." Pike obliged, placing Vicente alongside the open passenger's door.

"Ruthy, why don't ya' take our cutie here and plunk her down in the back seat. We'll make this comfortable for ya', babe."

"Don't do me any favors you slime ball," shouted Rita, who refused to let Ruth touch her. She walked over to the GTO and hesitated, not wanting to be confined in the back seat.

"Get in," said Farrell. Rita stayed put so Farrell said,

"Fine, have it your way."

Eli saw Ruth and Pike exchange looks. Pike nodded to Vicente that they were ready. Farrell drew his weapon and said, "Sorry folks, nothin' personal." He chambered a round and pointed the gun at Eli.

Chapter 28

The first shot is always the most startling. Everything is relatively quiet and then the peace is shattered by the loud report of the gun going off. No matter how many times Eli had been the unlucky participant in a shootout, his reaction was always the same. The sheer volume of it makes your ears ring, and the uncontrolled nature of it is distracting to the point of disorientation for those who've never been involved.

Eli instinctively convulsed into a crouch when the first round was fired. Agent Hunter yelled and fell sideways onto the ground in front of the GTO, his left arm fractured above the elbow by Pike's shot. Vicente grabbed Rita, threw her into the passenger's seat and ducked behind the door as Farrell, wheeled around to see what had happened. He turned just in time to see Ruth's Glock pointed at his head.

"Nothin' personal," she said with a smile as she shot him.

Farrell flinched just an inch to his left and the 9 millimeter slug hit him in the upper right shoulder above his body armor. The force of impact spun him backwards but he stayed on his feet and had the presence of mind to come around firing. One of his errant shots hit Ruth in the left leg and she screamed and crumpled to the ground, firing back as she fell.

Pike moved over in perfect firing position and also began shooting at Farrell, who dropped to the ground and rolled around on the gravel trying to avoid being hit. Pike's attention should have been spent on his fellow agent, Hunter, who recovered enough composure to get off a shot at him while lying on the ground.

The bullet hit Pike in the right leg and dropped him on his left side. He grabbed the wound with his gun hand as well as his free hand, and that was his second and final mistake. Hunter fired three more times in rapid succession, with two of the rounds hitting Pike's body armor. One bullet, however, got through his armor at the torso gap just under his right arm, and he dropped his pistol. His head lolled back against the gravel and he stopped moving.

Ruth had crawled back to the cover of the van and shot at Hunter from behind the right rear tire. Her first round was a lucky shot and hit Hunter in the top of the head, splattering his brains against the front bumper of the car. She propped herself up against the right rear wheel and looked back for Farrell.

Farrell had meanwhile worked his way to the back of the car and fired several more times at Ruth, striking the van but missing her. Eli slid out carefully and took Hunter's Glock from his limp right hand. He quickly dumped and checked the magazine to confirm how many rounds he had available, then drew back the slide and peered around the front of the car.

Vicente had pushed Rita into the back seat where she did not want to be, got in and closed the passenger door. Eli looked at him quickly through the open driver's door and Vicente nodded, letting Eli know that he and Rita were Ok.

Both agents had stopped firing, possibly to reload and Eli chanced another look around the car. Pike had rolled over onto his left side, so he was obviously still alive but not doing too well. Hunter was clearly dead and Ruth was badly wounded, likely bleeding out behind the van. Eli knew that Farrell had been hit at least once, but couldn't risk taking a look around the back of the car.

"Ruthy," yelled Farrell hoarsely. "Ruthy, how are ya' doing?"

"Oh, Ok," she gasped in reply. "Pretty messed up I guess. You got me good, Rick."

"Yeah, me, too," he answered. "Ruthy, you're gonna' bleed out unless ya' let me help ya'."

"Why would I do that, Rick? You want me dead, don't you?"

"I'm just trying to defend myself. You're the one who shot me first." He paused for a second and added, "If it's about the money, I know we can work somethin' out. Anyway, it looks like we have two extra shares to split up. We can work somethin' out."

Ruth moaned loudly and Eli saw Farrell stand up slowly and start gingerly walking towards the van.

"How do I know I can trust you, Rick?"

Farrell extended his weapon and walked slowly towards the back of the van. "How long we worked together, Ruthy? Two years? When have I ever steered ya' wrong? Trust me, I can help ya' but ya' gotta' let me come in now."

"Ok, Rick" she gasped. "Ok."

Eli peeked around the front of the car and watched as Farrell approached, his gun aimed straight ahead. *Bad move*, he thought.

Ruth dropped her pistol onto the ground and Farrell stepped into the clear where he could see her. He aimed carefully and slowly fired three rounds into her prostrate body, one into her body armor and two into her forehead. Eli saw her slump down against the wheel, dead on the gravel next to the van.

Pike moaned and attracted Farrell's attention back to the car. He turned and walked slowly over, and Eli could see only the non-fatal wound that Ruth had caused with her first shot. The rest of the bullets fired by Ruth and Pike had hit Farrell's body armor, and while they were solid hits, had left him with not much more than a few bad bruises and a cracked rib.

Farrell pointed his Glock at Pike and walked up to within two feet of him, intending to finish him off. Eli took aim and fired at Farrell and he fell backwards, screaming as he hit the gravel. He gasped and twisted on the ground and shot wildly into the air and in Eli's direction, but none of the bullets was even close.

Eli walked over to Farrell and grabbed his gun, tossing it back towards the van. He heard the faint sound of a helicopter coming their way and quickly realized it was Rodríguez and his men. In a few seconds they'd be there, and he had little time to get what he needed from Farrell. The young agent rolled from side to side and cursed the pain from the bullet Eli had put into his groin.

Eli grabbed Farrell's face with his free hand and shouted, "Where's the drop? Where are you meeting Paco?"

Farrell gasped, his face contorted in pain. "Biscayne National Park."

"When?"

"Tomorrow morning. Nine o'clock." Farrell gasped again and groaned loudly. "Ya' gotta' help me, please."

"Yeah, like you helped Ruth?"

"I'm dying here," moaned Farrell.

"Not hardly," said Eli angrily. He let Farrell go and walked back to the GTO.

"Vicente, it's clear," he called out. He put the Glock on the hood of his car and leaned against the passenger's side fender. Vicente got out and helped Rita from the back seat. She hugged him and then Eli and gasped when she saw the carnage.

"Is too bad," said Vicente quietly.

"They got what they deserved," said Rita, almost spitting the words out.

The helicopter landed about twenty feet from them and they had to shield their eyes from the cloud of lime dust kicked up by the rotors. The sound of police sirens soon mixed with the whine of the helicopter's turbine as a convoy of Miami Dade squad cars and unmarked FBI vehicles roared down the gravel road and stopped behind them.

Just as before, Rodríguez came running out of the helicopter and stopped when he saw the scene in front of him. Eli, Rita, and Vicente raised their hands as the police encircled them, but Rodríguez waved his men off and walked over to Eli. Paramedics raced to attend to Farrell and Pike, and checked Ruth and Hunter for signs of life.

"Don't say it," said Rodríguez with a loud sigh.

"Say what?" said Eli.

"You were right. This was too risky, and I should have known it was Farrell. I didn't think they could get away from us but I was wrong. I'm sorry."

"I thought you must have at least suspected someone when the bust in Mexico fell apart," said Eli sympathetically. "I was hoping not to be turned into bait so you could flush them out, but it worked out Ok for us."

"Not so good for them," added Vicente.

Rodríguez shook his head.

"You do everything you can to make things work, but for some people it's never enough. I promoted that SOB over a dozen other agents and he could care less. Hey, how is she?" Rodríguez called out to the paramedics attending to Ruth and one of them shook his head.

"Damn it! One corrupt SOB is all it takes to wipe out a promising group of agents. I should have seen it."

"Go easy on yourself," said Eli, patting him on the shoulder. "They were all adults. They knew what they were doing was wrong and the risks they were taking working for the cartels. They made a choice - a bad one, but it was their choice, not yours."

Rodríguez smiled faintly. "You're all Ok?"

Rita nodded but stayed tucked between Eli and Vicente.

"If I hadn't got a call from Bill Sexton at the *Herald* we might never have found you. Seems someone tipped him to the meet at the river and he saw the whole thing go down. A real fortunate coincidence, don't you think?"

Eli smiled dryly but said nothing.

"I'll need statements from all of you tomorrow, but you can go for now. Be at my office at nine tomorrow morning." The agent turned to go but Eli held his arm.

"Well, we can't make that time," Eli said slowly. "You see, Paco is going to make the drop for this job at Biscayne National Park tomorrow at nine. I'm sick and tired of being set up and I want to finish this guy, once and for all. I've got a plan but I need your cooperation. How would you like to join us?"

Rodríguez contemplated the opportunity for a few seconds and then smiled. "Ok, let's try it your way this time. What have you got in mind?"

§

Sundays in South Florida seem to start slower than they do in other parts of the country. This is especially true in the summer, when the air can be dead still and you can actually *see* the humidity in the air. On days like this there are only four places to be: at church, at the beach, playing dominoes with your friends, or having breakfast at your favorite air conditioned restaurant. There are loads of others of course, but for Eli and Vicente those four pretty much characterized their Sundays every June, July, and August.

Unfortunately, they were not destined for any of

those activities this Sunday morning. Instead, they once again found themselves in the white panel van headed for the marina parking lot of Biscayne National Park sharing the space with an FBI SWAT team in full body armor. Not exactly the typical group they would choose to socialize with on a Sunday, but for sure a good group to have on your side.

Determined not to be outgunned by the drug smugglers, each member of the team carried an H&K MP5K light machine gun with four thirty-two round clips and a Glock 22 in a side holster. Eli rode in the back with the team but planned to sit this one out. Vicente, however, rode in the front with Rodríguez, who had insisted on directing this operation from the ground.

The van arrived in the parking lot precisely at nine in the morning and proceeded to the back set of docks nearest the bay. Vicente and Rodríguez could see two Chevy Suburbans and a black Mercedes parked near one of the docks as they approached, proof that Paco had already checked the area and was awaiting their arrival. Upon seeing the van enter the parking area, Paco's men clambered out of their SUV's and stood in front of the Mercedes. They kept their guns concealed for the moment so as not to cause too much of a stir with the local fishermen.

Rodríguez drove the van to within a few yards of the waiting group and stopped with the vehicle pointed forward.

"Ok Vicente, remember the plan and do as I say. Understand?"

"*Si, amigo.* Don worry. Is my day off." The old man smiled and Rodríguez flashed a grin before he got out of the van.

Vicente got out of the passenger's side and Rodríguez walked behind him with his Glock pointed at Vicente's back. They walked slowly towards the Mercedes and Paco's men drew their weapons as a precaution. Paco and one of his bodyguards got out of the car with another briefcase and walked forward a few feet to get a good look at what was happening. He pulled down his sunglasses and stared at Vicente as if he couldn't believe what he saw.

"What the fuck is this? Where's Farrell?" he shouted.

"There's been a change in plans," yelled Rodríguez. "Farrell couldn't make it. He's going to be away for awhile. I'm running things now."

"What the hell is this guy doing here?" shouted Paco, waving at Vicente. "I had a deal with Farrell, and this wasn't it."

"That's why Farrell won't be around anymore. He took too many chances, and I'm not him. I have the guy, but I'm not cleaning up your mess. He's your problem, so you deal with him. You contact me for the other stuff, the same way you did Farrell. That's the new deal, as of today. Let's have the money."

Paco ran his hands through his hair and stared at the pavement. "Screw this," he said.

"The deal's off."

Just as Paco turned to leave Rodríguez said, "Take him down," into the microphone under his shirt. The back doors of the van burst open and the SWAT team ran forward in two groups to encircle Paco and his guards. One of his men raised his weapon to fire but was quickly killed by a burst from one of the MP5's.

Paco ran like a gazelle down the dock towards a speed boat that had just started its engines. He jumped in and the boat shot off towards the entrance to Biscayne Bay.

"Not this time, asshole," said Rodríguez. "He's coming out," he shouted into his microphone again. "Get him and bring him back here." Just as he said that, two large DEA pursuit boats sped in from the bay and blocked the channel, stopping Paco's escape plan almost before it started. The agents in the boats drew their weapons on Paco and the driver, who raised their hands while the agents boarded them. They towed the boat back towards the dock with the dour-looking Paco, hands behind his back in handcuffs.

After the guard had been shot by the SWAT team the rest of Paco's men surrendered and laid down on their stomachs with their weapons at their sides. The SWAT team members quickly scooped up their guns and began to handcuff all of them as they lay on the pavement. Vicente embraced Rodríguez and gave him an emphatic hug. Finally, the longest two weeks of his life were coming to a close.

Eli walked over and shook the Special Agent's hand. "Great job, Rodríguez. I'm really happy to see that we finally got him."

"Yes, I'm sure you are. It's a relief for us, too. It's been a long and bloody battle."

Several smaller unmarked FBI vans and Crown Victoria's entered the parking area and drove up to them, ready to transport Paco and his men to a federal holding facility in downtown Miami. Paco was marched back up the dock by the DEA agents and crossed in front of Eli, Vicente, and Rodríguez on his way to one of the vans.

"I'll get you bastards, just wait. I'll get you. You're all dead, all of you. You're dead!" he yelled, spit flying from his mouth.

The trio stared at him and said nothing in reply, and his DEA escort shoved him hard in the back towards the vans. Paco stumbled to his knees and got up slowly, then the agents grabbed him by the arms and dragged him the rest of the way to the vans.

Vicente smiled. "He no very happy. Is possible he can be free?"

"Not a chance," said Rodríguez. "We've got him dead to rights. With your testimony, plus Farrell's and Pike's we should be able to put him away for a couple hundred years."

"So your guys agreed to testify?" asked Eli.

The young agent frowned. "Farrell will cut a deal to avoid the death penalty, and Pike will do the same when he recovers. I'm pretty certain of that."

Eli let out a deep sigh and relaxed for the first time in two weeks. "So it's finally over?"

"Yes, it's finally over," said Rodríguez. "Thanks to you guys, we were able to jump the investigation ahead by months and finally nail this guy on something concrete. We brought down the organization in Miami and cut off at least one source of drugs to the Mexican cartels. I'd say it's been a good couple of weeks."

Vicente looked at Eli and hugged him, patting his back. "*Amigo*, we are free. We can go now?"

"You owe me some paper work first," said Rodríguez. "I'll give you a ride to the office and we should be able to wrap everything up in a couple of hours. Your cars are there anyway, guys. The surveillance team removed the tracking transponder from your car yesterday, Vicente, so that's where it is now, in our secure garage."

"Great. Ok, then, let's get this over with." Eli put his arm around his old mentor's shoulder and they followed Rodríguez to one of the unmarked Crown Victoria's that had arrived with the vans. They met Rita as she got out of one of the Crown Vic's. She had been kept safely out of the action by the second group of agents and only now felt safe enough to show herself.

"By the way," said Eli as they all got into the car, "what's your first name? Or do you just want to be known as "Rodríguez" for the rest of your life?"

The agent laughed as he drove back out of the park, his companions beside and behind him.

"You know what they say - you can call me whatever you want, but my *mama* calls me Orlando."

"Is a good name, Orlando," said Vicente.

"Ok, so Orlando it is. I like Orlando, *Disney World* and all that. Maybe we should nickname you "Diz." Eli looked at him from the passenger's seat and grinned.

"Rodríguez will do just fine," said the agent.

They drove back downtown and rode the elevator up to the task force office, which Vicente was pleased to finally see.

"Last time I am here was no very much fun," he reminded the young agent.

"Yes, I know. Sorry about that, but we didn't know who you were at the time, and we had to be careful."

The lights were off in all but a few offices and most of the task force members were either at the bust or working out logistics of the prisoner transfers to the holding facility. Rodríguez turned on the light in his cluttered office and pulled two extra chairs in from the adjacent office.

"Ok, folks, take a seat. We need to check some boxes and fill in some blanks."

They sat there and cooperated with the questions and the tedium of the forms, which took four hours to complete.

"The federal prosecutor will want to talk to all three of you sometime next week, so don't plan any long trips." The young agent smiled and added, "Go home and get some rest. I'll be in touch. I'll call the garage and tell them to release your cars to you. I'll do that paperwork so don't worry."

"Thanks for everything," said Eli. He and Vicente shook hands with Rodríguez and Rita smiled limply, and they took the elevator down to the garage to claim their vehicles. The guard checked their driver's licenses and then handed over the keys to the weary group.

"I'll take Rita home," Eli volunteered. "Take Monday off and then plan on coming to the office on Tuesday so we can wrap up our own reports."

"Ok, Eli. I see you Tuesday." Vicente hugged Rita, got into the big Corvette and roared out of the garage.

Eli and Rita followed Vicente out of the garage and headed down 7th Street towards Rita's condo. He glanced over to tell her something but stopped himself when he saw she was sound asleep, leaning back against the headrest. He smiled and continued on, rubbing his eyes and face to fight off his own exhaustion and sense of relief.

He had to shake her shoulder hard when they arrived at her building to get her to wake up.

"Rita, we're here. You Ok?"

"Yeah, boss, I'm Ok," she said stretching and looking around.

"You want me to walk you up?"

"No, I'm Ok. Thanks for everything, Eli. I knew you and Vicente would find a way to get me out of that shit."

"Well, it was a pretty close call. I'm really sorry about everything. We never should have put you in that situation to begin with." He held her hand and she smiled.

"I'm the one that's sorry. I should have listened to you in the first place and gone to see my sister, but I just wanted to help."

"Hush," said Eli. "don't worry about it. Go get a decent night's sleep and let this pass. Everything will be fine now."

"I never doubted you for a minute," she replied with a yawn. She leaned over and kissed him on the cheek. "See you on Tuesday."

Eli could only smile and watch as Rita dragged herself through the door and into the main lobby. He stared through the glass to watch as she got into the elevator and drove away only after the doors closed. He decided to head back to the office to check for any telephone messages and to straighten the place up a bit more before they started back to work on Tuesday. He saw the message light flashing when he entered and went over to Rita's desk to play the messages.

"You have.......two.......new.......messages," said the machine. "First message, received Saturday, nine PM."

"Eli, it's Bill Sexton. I hope you're still alive and are the one playing this message. Just wanted to thank you for the tip and I hope that Rodríguez found you in time. If not, I'll be at your funeral. If he did, you owe me a beer at least. Call me on Monday - please."

Eli smiled and vowed to take his old friend out for a nice dinner.

"Next message, received today, ten AM."

"Eli, it's Jo. I'd like to see you. Please call me as soon as you can."

He replayed Jo's message three times, trying to interpret some hint of purpose or emotion in it but he was too tired to tell. It would have to wait until he'd slept.

He closed up the office and dragged himself back to his car, driving the short distance to his condo in only a few minutes. He walked slowly to his bedroom once he'd entered his flat and just fell into bed without undressing.

That's where he was when he heard a loud ringing in his ears, seemingly only a few minutes later. Eli pried his eyes open and glanced over at his alarm clock. Light streamed in from the curtains and he could see it was after ten in the morning, and the ringing in his ears was from the telephone, which continued unabated.

"Ok, Ok," he said aloud, reaching for the receiver. "Yeah, this is Eli," he said hoarsely.

"Eli, it's Jo. Can you come over today? I need to talk to you about a few things."

He woke up and rolled over on his back.

"Sure, Jo. When do you want to see me?"

"How about noon? We'll have lunch. I have a lot to tell you." She sounded excited and her enthusiasm refreshed Eli a bit.

"I'll be there," he said, hanging up the phone.

Chapter 29

Eli rolled off the bed and stripped as he entered the bathroom. He showered, shaved and changed into his good Armani trousers and white shirt. His feet were killing him so he slipped on his clean Sperry Topsider's and left for the McHenry estate.

When he arrived he was surprised to see a girl open the door. She was about twenty with closely cut hair and wore beige pants and a matching jacket. Her appearance was striking and surprising to Eli, who expected the grumpy butler from his previous visit. Her fine facial features were set off by bright red lipstick and dark liner that emphasized her large brown eyes.

Eli was momentarily dumbstruck and just stared at the girl when she greeted him.

"Yes, can I help you?" she said with a beguiling smile.

He cleared his throat and said, "Yes. Um, I'm here to see Jo McHenry. She's expecting me."

"You must be Mr. Rose," the girl said. "I am Elena. Please follow me."

Eli went in and followed Elena to the patio where

he saw Jo, sitting at a table under a large umbrella. Elena smiled again and extended her hand towards Jo, then left.

It was a little bit windy, and Jo's hair blew around and partially covered her sunglasses. It was much shorter now, a slightly longer version of the "pixie" cut that was popular with younger people. It was apparently a concession to her new position as a company executive, and Jo did look a bit more conservative but no less sexy. She wore a loose white skirt and a white bikini top which set off her dark tan against the bright blue water of the bay. She stared down at some papers on the table and didn't immediately notice as Eli walked up.

"Hi, Jo," he said.

"Eli!" Jo jumped up from her chair and grabbed him, hugging him tightly for what seemed like a full minute.

"I missed you," she said with a long stare and a smile. "Please sit. I have so much to tell you."

"I see there have been some changes here."

Jo smiled. "I did tell you that I'd make some changes if it was up to me, and since it is up to me now, that's what I've done."

Eli surveyed the grounds but noticed only a few cosmetic changes, like the new patio furniture and, of course, the new staff.

"I like the direction you've taken with the staff."

"I'm sure you do," said Jo. "And Elena's not the only change. I have a new chef as well, and the house maids are also new. It's time the place moved out of the 1970's and into the 1990's."

"You're looking rested," he said, glancing at her legs as if for the first time.

"I am, but it's a stressful time now with the company in transition. Eli, I want to explain to you what's happened with the company, about where I am now and how my life will be for awhile."

He felt his stomach drop like he'd been punched. *Here it comes again*, he thought. *Another kiss off.*

"Sure, Jo. But you don't have to explain anything to me. After all, I'm only an employee, and I think we're all settled up on our accounts."

Jo frowned but was interrupted by her new chef, Raul.

"*Señorita*, would you like me to begin the service now that your guest has arrived?"

"Yes, please," she answered, and Raul bowed and smiled as he walked off towards the kitchen.

"As I was saying, I *want* to explain what's going on because I feel I owe you that. When we parted company I felt like there was some tension between us, and I don't want that."

Eli sat silently and looked at the girl, admiring her beauty as he did the very first time he'd seen her. She took off her sunglasses and put them on the table on top of her paperwork. He could see the pained expression in her eyes, something she clearly wanted him to see.

"Eli, I know I was supposed to call you a week ago, but things have been pretty crazy. I'm sorry I didn't call."

"Don't worry about it," he replied. "I was kind of tied up until yesterday, so I couldn't have done much anyway."

Jo eyed him curiously and knew there was something he wasn't telling her.

"I see. Well anyway, we had a special Board of Directors meeting on Saturday. The Board voted to appoint me Chairman - or Chairwoman - in Father's place and they are going along with my plan to reorganize the company. Lloyd stepped down as a result and has decided to leave the company."

"Congratulations. That's everything you wanted. I'm very happy for you."

He'd thought for a long time about what he was going to say next, mulling it over in his mind on the drive over. He decided to broach the subject anyway, knowing it would likely forma wedge between them, but he had to know.

"So, did you accept the money from Durán?"

She frowned but nodded, and Eli shook his head, feeling sad and disappointed.

"Eli, you have to understand. I had no choice. I had to bring something to the Board or they would have thrown me out without even allowing me to state my case. Manuel did what he said he would – he had the money wired when we were still in Trinidad so it was already in my Cayman Islands account when we got back to Miami. When I was able to bring forward one hundred fifty million dollars and a business plan that utilized the cash in a smart way the Board immediately threw their support behind me. Lloyd wasn't able to offer anything, so in the end there really was no contest. The money was the critical piece that let me regain control. Without it I'd be out of my own company, my family's company. I couldn't let that happen, not even if the funds came from a questionable source."

"A questionable source?" said Eli, surprised at his own anger. Just then Raul re-appeared with Elena, who held a large tray of plates adorned with various small portions of seafood.

"Pardon me," he said politely. "We have a trio of small dishes for you to try. Here, a West Indian-style curry of shrimp and fish, here, some pan-seared East Coast scallops, and here, Yucatán-style grouper. I've selected a nice Pinot Grigio for you today. Please enjoy." He smiled as Elena placed the plates on the table, then they left and returned to the kitchen.

Jo put her head in her hands and looked down at the pool deck. "Eli, I....."

"Questionable sources, eh?" repeated Eli. "That's an understatement if I've ever heard one. You know exactly where Durán got the money. You know how dirty it was, how dirty he was. That was blood money in the truest sense."

"Eli, I had no choice."

"You always have a choice," he said softly. "So far the good thing for you is that the guy that funded you won't be around to ask for payment, but there's no guarantee his bosses won't come looking for the money someday. It's a pretty clean deal right now, but I don't think you will ever be able to rest easily knowing the source."

Jo looked out at the bay, shook her head and sighed.

"I knew the risks and I explained why I did what I did. I don't expect you to understand, but I wanted to explain it to you anyway. Maybe I hoped you'd understand." She reached her hand across the table and squeezed his hand tightly.

Eli's anger subsided into a deep sadness and sense of loss. He actually did understand all too well how such things can happen. How sometimes, people make choices they have to make for a number of reasons that may not seem so clear to others. He understood how sometimes you can feel like you are backed into a corner and you have no choice but to act in the best way you can at the time. He'd been through that himself, he'd *lived* it. But that understanding didn't take the sting out of it for him, knowing she'd compromised her morals for the money and the power that went with it.

"I know you did what you thought you had to do." He squeezed her hand and then let it go.

"So that's it?" she said, her voice quivering with emotion.

"That's it," he lied.

His own moral compass was very clear on what had happened, even if Jo's wasn't. Knowing what she'd done was a deal breaker for him, and although he didn't like the thought of judging her, he couldn't help himself in the end.

"Let's leave it like this," he began. "You're a busy person with a company to run, and I'm just a beat up old guy that runs a lost and found office. We're moving in two completely different orbits that just happened to cross for a few weeks this summer."

That seemed easier to him than confronting her with his true feelings. He'd taken the easy way out and was conflicted about it, but he cared for her so much he just couldn't bring himself to tell her how he really felt. Eli got up to leave but she grabbed his hand again to keep him from going.

Tears began to stream down Jo's face as she stood up beside him. "Please Eli. It doesn't have to be like this. We can just go on like before."

"You know things can't be like they were in the Bahamas. That was paradise for me, but in the end it wasn't real. We both know that. This," he said choking back his own emotions, "this place, your life, what you've done, all this is what's real. It's not my life and you know it never can be."

She put her head on his shoulder and sobbed. She hugged him and nodded, knowing he was right.

"You'll do great running your company," Eli added. "You've got the drive, the talent. You'll do great."

Jo looked up at him and nodded. Eli held her back at arm's length and then kissed her one last time.

"Like Bogey said to Bergman, Here's looking at you, kid."

Jo broke down and hugged him again and then let him go. Eli turned and walked back through the house and let himself out without turning around to look at her. He felt sick to his stomach and his knees were weak and wobbly, and he knew that if he turned to look he might not leave, even though he had to.

He drove back to his office and parked his car in the garage, but he didn't go straight up. Instead, he sat in the car with the windows open and let the breeze blow through for a few minutes. Eli hadn't really cried since his father passed away, but he sure felt like crying now. He needed to regain his composure and clear his head.

Why do I always end up with these women I can't

hang onto? he thought. *There has to be something wrong with me.* He shook his head and felt very sad. Then he closed up the GTO, and walked off towards the elevators

§

"I didn't look at any of these before we left. Maybe you want to read them?" Eli handed the small stack of newspapers to Vicente, who had to grab them with both hands to keep them from blowing overboard.

"*Si*, of course, *amigo*. Is very interesting to me."

Vicente held one front page section up and stowed the other papers below in the cabin. The boat rocked a bit in the waves but was otherwise steady and Eli had her tacking into the wind at a good rate.

"I'm glad you agreed to come with me," said Eli, yelling into the wind. "I know sailboats aren't your favorite means of transport."

"I no will miss this," Vicente yelled back. "But you say the last time that you take me on vacation when we finish the case, so this is Ok with me."

Eli smiled and stared out at the horizon. He steered the big Out Islander southwest but wasn't really too concerned about the time. They'd set off from Nassau at first light and they should have enough light, even at seven in the evening to see the island, so he was relaxed and felt that way for the first time in months.

This was indeed the vacation Eli had promised Vicente when they first accepted the job from Jo McHenry. It took a few months, but now that all the legal issues were behind them they were free to leave the country for as long as they wished.

"I wish Rita had changed her mind," said Eli.

"Yes, is a shame." Vicente was practicing his English again and Eli was impressed and encouraging when he could be. He knew that Vicente wanted to keep it low-key but he also knew that Vicente was proud of his progress.

Vicente looked over the paper and smiled.

"It say here that Paco has a deal with the government. Look." He held the paper up so Eli could read the headline.

"Gutiérrez cuts a deal with federal prosecutors," said Eli aloud. He read on. ".....will avoid prosecution on drug charges by cooperating and agreeing to testify against major Colombian and Mexican cartel members." Eli paused. "Wow, that guy has nine lives," he exclaimed.

Vicente waved up at him in agreement. After the US attorney presented the sworn depositions of Eli, Vicente, and Rita to Paco's lawyer, Paco decided to cooperate and try for a plea bargain in return for immunity from prosecution. At the same time, Rodríguez convinced Pike to testify against Farrell in Ruth's killing, so with everything wrapped up he was a happy man when he was offered and accepted a transfer to Washington.

Eli noticed that the story was written by Bill Sexton, and he was glad to see in a separate article that he'd been nominated for a Pulitzer Prize for his investigative reporting on the link between the cartels. Thankfully for Eli and Jo, Bill didn't continue his research into the connection between Paco Gutiérrez and the McHenrys because it now looked like a dead-end. With Donald McHenry missing and presumed dead and Paco singing like a bird in federal custody there wasn't much of a story left. He'd made his big score with the Colombian and Mexican cartel connection, and that's where he'd decided to invest the majority of his investigative efforts.

Eli was happy that Bill's lack of interest spared Jo any further suffering, which also meant that she didn't have the cocaine scandal hanging over her head when she needed all the help she could get with the re-launch of the McHenry Group (now minus Lloyd Taylor). Her parents could rest in peace and she could get on with her life.

Eli felt a twinge of nostalgia as the Joulters Cays came into view on the horizon, but it was only a minor twinge, or at least it started that way. It clearly wasn't the same without Jo at the wheel of the *Bree-zee*, hair blowing across her tanned, smiling face. The twinge grew and pulled at his gut, surprising him and darkening his mood. He cast a stare at the cabin, half expecting to hear her call out to him, but then shook his head and focused on the rapidly approaching islands again.

No, Jo was gone from his life, likely for good, and the *Bree-zee* was still in dry dock, getting her keel refitted and her bottom painted after the beating she'd suffered on the beach. His intuition and personal sense of right and wrong had cost him a lot, but that's how things work out sometimes.

The money from the case had finally provided him with a sense of independence and freedom he hadn't felt since before his father died. Plus, his relationships with Vicente and Rita and his friends were stronger than ever. *Small price to pay*, he mused to himself. A dinner for Bill, another for Leslie, and a sailing vacation for Vicente. Rita was off playing Auntie to her sister's kids in Orlando, all expenses paid. They all seemed pretty pleased. And Jo – even though she was on her own and headed for success, the cost to her soul was terrible and unrecoverable. That part was the agonizingly sad part for Eli. Still, there was one last thing left undone.

"Hey, old man. Come up here and lend a hand on the lines."

Vicente obliged and they lowered and stowed the sails and motored into shallow water near the south part of the main island. The sun was low on the horizon and shadows from the tree-lined dunes stretched out across the water to blanket their boat, but Eli was determined to fulfill his final obligations before the sun went down that day. Vicente helped him lower the small dingy into the water and Eli cranked up the motor and sped off towards the island.

He ran the boat onto the beach and brought the bowline with him to the trees. He tied it off around a fallen pine and slogged up the beach with his heavy duffle bag. Just above the storm high tide line he squatted on his knees and removed the large bronze plaque from the bag. He nailed the plaque to the sturdiest tree he could find and sat back to admire his work.

"Ok, Jo. Just for you," he said wistfully, butterflies in his stomach.

He cleared his throat as if he were about to give a speech to an audience and said, "In loving memory of Donald and Madeleine McHenry. May the wind fill your sails and the seas comfort your souls. Your loving daughter, Jo."

That was her final request of him a few weeks ago and he couldn't refuse her this final gesture. After all, Jo had nowhere else to mark her parents passing, and the island sure seemed like the most fitting place to do it.

Eli got up and walked a short distance down the beach until he could see the place where he'd left the Beretta. It was still wrapped in his handkerchief and wasn't too badly corroded by the salt air. *Hello old friend*, he said to himself. *With a little cleaning you'll be as good as new*. He ran back to the dingy as the last rays of sunlight began to disappear below the silhouette of the island and motored back to the boat.

"Eli, I have prepare some food. Where have you been for so long?" Vicente seemed concerned but not too bothered.

"Just fulfilling a final obligation and cleaning up the beach a bit," he replied. "What did you make for us?"

"Ah, we have some *croquetas* of *mero* - oh, I am sorry. Some croquettes of grouper with onion and spices." Vicente seemed pleased he was able to correct himself and do the English translation.

"Also I have good Cuban garlic bread and we have some beer. How this sounds to you?"

"Excellent, my friend. Tomorrow we'll do some fishing and then head back. What do you think?"

"This is great, Eli. This is great."

Epilogue

Rita yawned as she rode the elevator up to the office. She was happy to be back but had become accustomed to sleeping past six in the morning while she was visiting her sister. She struggled a bit more with her large purse than usual, maybe because she was restocking her work space with the tissues and other things she kept close by. With the heavy purse slung over her left shoulder she had one hand free to carry her plastic lunch cooler in the other, but she still had to struggle with the keys to the office.

She opened the door and immediately noticed that the lights were on. A jolt of fear shot down her spine as she suddenly remembered the moment Paco's men had burst in on her and taken her away at gunpoint. Rita was afraid until she smelled coffee and saw that the lights in Eli's office were also on.

"Wow, what are you doing here?" She stood by the door and was astonished to see her boss at his desk. It was the first time in their entire working relationship that she'd ever seen him arrive first, yet there he was, reading the sports section of the *Miami Herald* and drinking his coffee.

"What do you mean?" said Eli. "This is my office. Why shouldn't I be here?"

"You know what I'm talking about. You're never here this early. What's going on?"

"Nothing," Eli lied. "Just wanted to see your smiling face and find out how your visit to your sister's place went."

Rita eyed Eli suspiciously as she pulled things from her purse. She turned on her computer and went into his office and sat down.

"Oh, it was a great visit. We had a great time. Thanks again for paying for everything. You didn't have to do that."

"It was the least I could do for you," said Eli with his head buried in the paper. "You deserve more."

Rita grabbed the paper and said, "Ok, Eli. What the hell's going on? I know you're up to something, so better you tell me now or else."

Eli grabbed the paper back and glared at her. "Or else what?"

The hot *Latina* leaned forward onto his desk so that her large breasts swung low and nearly popped out of her blouse. She swayed back and forth on purpose, just enough for them to move tantalizingly close to Eli's face and tease him unmercifully.

"Or else I'll have to *make* you tell me what's going on."

Eli was transfixed on her chest for a moment but quickly regained his composure.

"Rita, nothing's going on. Everything is fine."

She stood up and walked over next to him, so close

he could feel his heartbeat race. She could always get him to cooperate when she teased him like she did in the old days, and he was still a sucker for her ample charms.

"Really, Eli? There's nothing you want to tell me?"

Eli gulped and tried to look away from her. He'd promised to stay away and go slow, but this didn't seem that way to him. Still, he knew she wouldn't stop until he confessed, so now in a decidedly weakened state, he knew he was beaten.

"Well, there is this one thing."

"Ha!" she shouted. "I knew it! What are you keeping from me? You know, every time you do this it only makes everything more difficult."

"Ok, Ok. Jim's on his way over."

"Jim Morgan? Are you serious? Why is he coming here?" Rita now stood back several feet, clearly angry.

"He wants to talk about a job. I thought I owed it to him to hear what he had to say, especially since he bailed me out of Trinidad last year."

Rita began to curse in Spanish, a long string of words that Eli could mostly make out and didn't like much.

"Eli, you don't need this anymore. You don't have to work for this guy if you don't want to."

"I know that. But you know me, Rita. I can't just quit cold turkey. You know how I am."

The little red head put her hands on her round hips and shook her head.

"You are some piece of work, Eli Rose. But I do know you pretty well, and I know you need this." She walked over to him and gave him a hug, smothering his face against her cleavage.

"When is he supposed to be here?"

"Any minute now."

"Oh my gosh," she exclaimed in a panic. "I've got to leave right now. You know I can't be here when he gets here. He'll be all over me if I'm here. I'll call you in an hour to see if he's gone." She quickly gathered up her purse, grabbed a coffee and ran out with a wave and a smile.

Eli shook his head and laughed. He really missed her when they all went their separate ways for vacation, and he was looking forward to working with her again. He'd known Rita longer than any other woman and worked more closely with her than anyone else. He was Ok with their working relationship the way it was, but any time she wanted to change it he was all for it.

His mind wandered to thoughts of Rita when he heard the office door open again.

"Rita," he called out. "I need some more coffee."

"At your service, sweetheart," said Morgan, sticking his head into the office. "Mind if I come in?"

"Sure, Jim. How have you been?" They shook hands and Morgan sat down across the desk from his former employee.

"Ok. You know how it is up there."

"Yes, I remember. So what's on your mind? I know you didn't come all this way just to shoot the breeze for a half hour."

Morgan smiled and leaned back in his chair.

"Remember on our little trip back from Trinidad last year, how I told you 'bout a little problem we are havin' in Venezuela. Well, things ain't improved any, and I need some help sortin' it all out."

"Sortin' it out," Eli repeated. "Sounds like a familiar refrain to me. Just what does that mean, anyway?"

The older man smiled and stared hard at Eli. He knew he'd have to tell him everything this time, so he just opened the flood gates and let it all come out.

"Well, we've been cooperatin' with the "Vennies" the last couple of years, runnin' search and destroy missions along the Colombian frontier chasing down FARC cells and command structure. Last year when I first mentioned this to you, we'd just lost contact with one of our teams out there in the Sierra Perijá. Now it's happened again, this time in the area southwest of La Fría. We need a non-affiliated team to go down there and find out what happened to the teams and get our guys back, if that's possible. What do you think?"

"I think you're flipping crazy to be messing around down there. That whole area is like a free fire zone. You've got FARC, narco-traffickers, corrupt *Guardia Nacional*. Could you have picked a worse place?"

Morgan sighed and stroked his thin blond hair.

"Come on Eli, you know the drill. We're there because we have to be. Will you help us or not?"

Eli contemplated the situation and wasn't sure.

"What kind of support is available?"

"You mean military support?" said Morgan with surprise.

"If I get into trouble down there, what kind of support will I have?" Eli pressed the point.

Morgan stared at Eli but relented. "You know how this works. Plausible deniability is the way of the world in Washington these days, so if you get yourself into some kind of trouble everyone will spout the line that you're just some crazy "Rambo" type playin' hero."

He sighed but looked Eli in the eyes and added, "But between you and me, if you need help you'll have it. Just don't put yourself in a position to need it. Our minders in Congress won't be happy if it ever comes out that we're doin' clandestine stuff on that border, and it will make my life a livin' hell. I still haven't come to the end of all that shit we caught for what happened in Nicaragua. The last thing I need is for somethin' like this to blow up in my face."

"Understood," said Eli flatly. "I'll try to keep your life as simple as possible. So here's the deal - double the usual fee, no arguments. All expenses paid, thirty percent up front, and I get to pick the team."

"What?" shouted Morgan, rising out of his chair. "That's highway robbery. We can't pay that, and there's no way you're doin' this without some of my people bein' involved.."

"That's fine," said Eli with a smile. "I don't need the work, so I guess I'll say thanks for coming. It was good to see you again." He offered his hand to Morgan but the agent turned away.

"Dammit, Eli. Now that you have money you're turnin' into a pain in ass to work with. I guess I can't use the patriotism speech either, huh?"

"Nope. You used that one too many times."

Morgan slammed his hand down on the desk and sat down again.

"Shit, Eli. I guess you're the one who has all the leverage. Ok, it's a deal." They shook hands and Eli produced a note pad and a pen.

"Great. Ok, let's start. I'm all ears."

Morgan kicked back and put his cowboy boots up on the front of Eli's desk.

"Well, a not so funny thing happened on the way to the FARC camp about this time last year. One of our patrols was out on a DEA spotter plane when they were lost from radar. We assumed they'd crashed in the mountains but when we received a ransom demand from the bad guys, we knew we had a problem. I want you to go down there and bring back whoever survived after the plane went down."

"Shit. That sounds too much like Nicaragua. I don't know."

Morgan leaned forward and opened his hands.

"Eli, you know you're our guy for things like this. Anything that happens in the jungle, we're gonna' call you. You have to say yes."

"Jim, I'm getting too old for this." Eli rubbed his face and felt the lines and the years like never before.

"Nonsense. How old are you now? Forty? Forty three?"

"I'm forty four and feeling like I'm sixty four. Every one of these jobs takes a toll."

"I get it, but this is what you do." Morgan sat back and folded his arms, staring hard at Eli.

"Morgan, how old were you when you stopped doing field work?" asked Eli.

"I was forty one," said Morgan. Why?"

Eli smiled. *What a funny coincidence*, he thought. "No reason. Never mind. Ok, so when do we start?"